Understanding Addiction and Evil: Finding Healing Through the 12 Steps and Spirituality.

By

I0468189

Kevin G Stephenson. M.Div, M.A, LPC-S, BCC.

Introduction

This workshop will provide a general overview of nature and impact of addictions. First, I will discuss a basic philosophy regarding humanity. Second, I will review some basic statistics of the economic effects of the drug trade that fuel addictions and its financial impact on the economy. Third, I will look at the destructive impact of addictions on the human family (men, women and children). Fourth we will look at the physiological impact addiction has on the human brain. Fifth we will look at the 12 Step Model as a philosophy and how it is utilized to treat addictions. Fifth, we will also examine the scriptural basis for its development. Sixth we will review Roman Catholic theology as a source of healing for the sufferer. Last, I will present a few case studies I have encountered.

Philosophical Foundations

Socrates

Lived approximately (470/469 – 399 BC)[1] was a classical Greek (Athenian) philosopher credited as one of the founders of Western philosophy. He developed the Socratic Technique which is an ancient Greek technique of asking a question(s) to arrive at the core or fundamental meaning of the issue at hand. It is the art of asking a question that leads to follow up question to clarify true meaning. It is the examination of key moral concepts such as the Good and Justice. It was first described by Plato in the *Socratic Dialogues*. To solve a problem, it would be broken down into a series of questions, the answers to which gradually distill the answer a person would seek

Plato

Lived approximately (428/427 or 424/423 – 348/347 BC) grew up in Greece. He was a primary student of Socrates. Plato developed his ideas from Socrates with the doctrine of the immortality of the soul. The body is the matter and the soul is its form. The soul or psyche provided guidance to the mortal matter or flesh. The immortal soul contained the intellect or mind. The soul also controls the rational functions, intelligence, moral courage and the appetites or affections. Irrational thoughts were assumed to be the products of the mortal body. Platonic Realism is the belief in universal truths, objects or forms. These truths are constant regardless of temporal circumstances. The soul is a spiritual substance neither created nor destroyed. It pre-existed the created human body and must infuse the human being.

Aristotle

 Lived approximately (384 – 322 BC). He was also a Greek philosopher. He studied Platonic philosophy. He viewed the human person as dual natured with an identified psyche or mind that animates the consciousness: the body and life. The soul is immaterial, spiritual and immortal in nature. The soul is the real substance of the human being. The soul is the source of all physical motion. The soul is the final cause or inward goal regulator of the human person. The soul is the intellectual and rational function of the individual.

Saint Augustine

Lived (November 354 – 28 August 430) North Africa and Carthage, Rome. Saint Augustine a 4th century Catholic Church Father, states the human being is a perfect unity of two substances: soul and body. He argued that the soul was created immortal by God for the human body. At the very moment of conception the soul is infused into the body. The soul possesses the faculty of the will or choice. At the moment of death the soul is separated from the human body and remains eternal. However, at the resurrection, the soul will be reunited with the body.

Saint Thomas Aquinas:

Lived (1225 – 7 March 1274) Sicily, Italy. Saint Thomas Aquinas: a Roman Catholic Doctor of the Church rediscovered Aristotle's writings and embraced his concepts of the primacy of the soul in regards to the body. He believe there is one God who is wholly simple, unique and absolute being. God is the ultimate source of all creation. I also believe that humankind is made up two substances matter and spiritual form. Even though our bodies are temporal in nature, we possess eternal souls that cannot die. (G.C. Berkouwer 1962)

Evil Defined

Evil, in a large sense, may be described as the sum of the opposition to that which is good. We know this through our experience in the world. These experiences go against the healthy desires and needs of individuals and societies. When this occurs among people it creates suffering and pain. Thus evil, from the point of view of human beings, should not exist. It is self-evident that the experience of evil is negative and not positive. It is the loss or deprivation of something necessary for perfection or the good. Evil is experience is three ways. Physical evil, Moral evil and metaphysical evil.

Physical evil includes all that causes harm to man, whether by bodily injury, by thwarting his natural desires, or by preventing the full development of his powers, either in the order of nature directly, or through the various social conditions under which mankind naturally exists. Physical evils experienced in nature may come in the forms of sickness, accident, death, etc. Also in the form of poverty, oppression, and imperfect social/economic/political systems. Mental suffering, such as anxiety, disappointment, and remorse, and the limitation of intelligence which prevents human beings from attaining to the full comprehension of their environment, are congenital forms of evil.

Moral **evil** is experienced when people freely choose to act against the moral order. These are acts of which the human conscience clearly disapproves. This does not cover people who may be ignorant or unable to comprehend moral behavior.

Metaphysical **evil** is the limitation experienced in the natural world/universe. The natural world includes the animal, vegetable kingdoms and the cosmos. This is seen when the natural world does not attain its full or ideal perfection or good. These limitations occurs from physical conditions, or sudden catastrophes.

http://www.newadvent.org/cathen/05649a.htm

What is your definition of evil?

Addictions Defined:

The Latin root for the addiction is addico, addicere, addixi, addictus. It is translated as something someone is bounded too or judged by. It is any compulsive, persistent, escalating pattern, craving type behavior that reduces quality of life and is characteristically self-defeating or self-destructive in nature. It is evidenced by repeated failures to stop the behavior. It has a strong emotional and physical component that creates a high level of distress if not fulfilled. Great harm is expressed and experienced within the individual, interpersonal relationships, families and the community.
http://www.asam.org/for-the-public/definition-of-addiction
http://www.aamft.org/imis15/content/consumer_updates/sexual_addiction.aspx

General Statistics on Addictions

- Nearly 23 million Americans—almost one in 10—are addicted to alcohol or other drugs.
- More than two-thirds of people with addiction abuse alcohol.

- The top three drugs causing addiction are marijuana, opioid (narcotic) pain relievers, and cocaine. http://www.helpguide.org/harvard/addiction_hijacks_brain.ht m
- Abuse of tobacco, alcohol, and illicit drugs is costly to our Nation, exacting over $600 billion annually in costs related to crime, lost work productivity and healthcare. 2013: http://www.drugabuse.gov/related-topics/trends-statistics.

The Financial Impact of Drug Addiction

Tobacco: Healthcare: $96 Billion. Overall: $193 Billion
Alcohol: Healthcare: $30 Billion. Overall: $235 Billion
Narcotics: Healthcare: $11 Billion. Overall: $193 Billion

Drug Trafficking in the United States

- $13 billion per year global in revenue. https://www.unodc.org/unodc/en/drug-trafficking/index.html
- 60% of the world's illegal drugs are consumed by American drug users. http://drugabuse.com/library/workplace-drug-abuse/

Drug Addiction Related to Prison Offenses.

- $1 trillion over 40 years has been spent on the war against drugs. However, the United States has the world's largest incarceration rate.
- 2.2 million Americans are in prison or jail for drug related offenses.
    More than half of federal prisoners are incarcerated for drug crimes in 2010, according to the Bureau of Justice Statistics,
- The number of people in federal prison for drug offenses spiked from 74,276 in 2000 to 97,472 in 2010, according to the U.S. Department of Justice. http://www.huffingtonpost.com/2013/04/08/drug-war-mass-incarceration_n_3034310.html

Divorce Rates and Addictions

- According to DUI.com, "Statistics on the positive correlation between domestic violence and addiction range from forty-four percent, according to the New Jersey Uniform Crime Report of 1989, to more than eighty percent in some research studies." http://www.dui.com/
- A 2007 study done by the Rand Corporation found that alcohol was the single most significant factor in early divorce among young couples. *http://www.divorcelawfirms.com/resources/divorce/divorce-children/the-link-between-addiction-divorce*

School Drop-out Rate and Addictions

- Combined 2002 to 2010 data show that nearly one in seven youths aged 16 to 18 (13.2 percent), or 12th grade aged youths, had dropped out of school.
- Substance use rates among 12th grade aged youths who had dropped out of school were higher than among those who were still in school; for example, 56.8 percent of dropouts were current cigarette users compared with 22.4 percent of those still in school.
- There is a pattern of higher illicit drug use rates among dropouts than those still in school. The stats are the same for both males and females, as well as for Whites, Hispanics, and Blacks; *http://www.samhsa.gov/data/2k13/NSDUH036/SR036Substance UseDropouts.htm*

Child Abuse and Addiction

- It is estimated that 9 percent of children in this country (6 million) live with at least one parent who abuses alcohol or other illicit drugs (Substance Abuse and Mental Health Services Administration [SAMHSA], 2003). Studies indicate that between one-third and two-thirds of child maltreatment cases involve substance use to some degree (HHS, 1999).

- 22,440 children receiving in-home services for maltreatment and 128,640 to 211,720 children in out-of-home care had a parent with a substance use disorder in 2004. In that same year, approximately 295,000 parents receiving treatment for substance use had one or more children removed by child protective services. https://www.childwelfare.gov/pubs/factsheets/parentalsubabuse.cfm#1
- Fetal alcohol spectrum disorders (FASD) are among the most well-known consequences, affecting an estimated 40,000 infants born each year. Oklahoma had almost 11,000 kids in state custody—mostly because of illicit drug issues. This is a continued crisis because there is a shortage of families willing to consider foster care.
- Alcoholism among adult children of EHOH abusers is five times the general population. This is most likely due to the emotional trauma of living with an ETOH parent (Asquith 2010).

Work Force Lost and Addiction

- Of all drug users, 74.8 percent are employed and active in the workplace. This means that 12.9 million individuals actively use drugs in the workforce, according to the Occupational Safety & Health Administration (OSHA). Using drugs impairs decision-making abilities as well as physically impairs people.
- 10 to 20 percent of American workers who die at work have a positive result when tested for drugs or alcohol. A study by OSHA states that the most dangerous occupations, such as mining and construction, also have the highest rates of drug use by their employees.

http://drugabuse.com/library/workplace-drug-abuse/

Addiction Terms

Alcoholism: Is the third largest health problem in the United States (following heart disease and cancer). 7% of Americans suffer from alcoholism. It is considered incurable, potentially fatal but highly treatable disorder. People most vulnerable to ETOH abuse are those who form compulsive-addictive behavior patterns easily compared to the general population.

A progressive compulsive-addictive illness: The continued use of ETOH or poly substance excessively in a way that damages one or more area of a person's life. The areas affected are mental, physical health, family life, social relationships, job and economic viability, creativity and spiritual wholeness. (Asquith, 2010).

Compulsive: Psychologically the desire to abuse ETOH or Poly Substance is driven at an unconscious level. To the degree a person reports being out of control with the substance abuse.

Addictive: It is a physiological adaptation of a person to the ETOH/Poly Sub that creates acute distress and intense cravings when the abuse stops.

Progressive: When an illness progresses in predicable stages and if not treated will result in irreversible dysfunction and eventually death. Increased dependence or loss of control can progress over a period of 5 to 15 years.

Problem Drinking: Is an all-inclusive term which can include non-addictive ETOH behavior. An example would be driving an automotive while under the influence of ETOH. Or engaging in self destructive behavior (unprotected sexual behavior or altercations with strangers) while under the influence of ETOH.

Chronic Alcoholism: an advanced stage in the illness where severe medical or psychiatric complications occur.

Steady Drinker with Binges: their heavy daily drinking is accented by occasional binges of several days or longer.

Periodic Alcoholic: This person is abstinent between binges.

Plateau Alcoholic: This person drinks continually but seldom seeks maximum intoxication or goes on binges.

Recreational Drunkenness: Were groups of people use ETOH to release their child sides to play.

Social Desperation Drunkenness: intoxication to anesthetize suffering from social discrimination and injustice (Native Americans).

High or Low Bottom Alcoholics: Is the degree of personal or social disintegration a person has to experience before they seek outside help for the addiction.

Low Bottom Alcoholic: generally refers to skid row, indigent **or** homeless person due to ETOH abuse.

Soil of Addiction: Usually includes psychological problems that are present prior to the person abusing and becoming dependent on ETOH. ETOH is often utilized for its psychological pain numbing effects.

Pre-Alcoholics: People who consistently struggle with and lack adequate coping skills for anxiety, guilt, and inner conflict.

Triggers: Alcoholism for some follows a significant tragedy, trauma or loss.

Causations (Asquith, 2010).

Sociocultural: Learned social and cultural behaviors may be a contributing factor. For example in Ireland and France there is a higher rate of ETOH abuse compared to other countries.

Spiritual: Religious anxiety, fear of death, meaninglessness, unresolved guilt may contribute to ETOH abuse. Spiritual ETOH can falsely serve as a spiritual transcendences. ETOH addiction may serve as a form of idolatry. Idolatry in the sense of making ETOH abuse a false absolute out of a substance that is not absolute (mutable). Healing would involve addressing the universal spiritual needs such as trust, healthy values, meaning, forgiveness and the development of virtues (May, 1988, 1991).

Sexual Addiction

- Nearly 12 million people report suffering from sexual addiction in the United States.
- Sexual addiction is a serious problem in which one engages in persistent and escalating patterns of sexual behavior despite increasing negative consequences to one's self or others.
- The body produces many hormones and neurotransmitters during sex that produce the same chemical "high" as drugs or alcohol.
- Sex addicts, like other addicts, often have a background of abuse (sexual, physical, emotional) and/or neglect, and family histories sprinkled with numerous addictions. http://www.aamft.org/imis15/content/consumer_updates/sexual_addiction.aspx

Human Sex Trafficking

- Human Sex trafficking generates $9.5 billion yearly in the United States. (United Nations)
- Approximately 300,000 children are at risk of being prostituted in the United States. (U.S. Department of Justice).
- The average age of entry into prostitution for a child victim in the United States is 13-14 years old. (U.S. Department of Justice).
- A pimp can make $150,000-$200,000 per child each year and the average pimp has 4 to 6 girls. (U.S. Justice Department, National Center for Missing and Exploited Children) .
- The average victim may be forced to have sex up to 20-48 times a day. (Polaris Project)

Eating Disorders

- Almost 50% of people with eating disorders meet the criteria for depression.
- Only 1 in 10 men and women with eating disorders receive treatment. Only 35% of people that receive treatment for eating disorders get treatment at a specialized facility for eating disorders.
- Up to 24 million people of all ages and genders suffer from an eating disorder (anorexia, bulimia and binge eating disorder) in the U.S.
- Eating disorders have the highest mortality rate of any mental illness. http://www.anad.org/get-information/about-eating-disorders/eating-disorders-statistics/

Carbohydrate (Glucose/Sugar) Addictions

- When people eat a food containing carbohydrates, the digestive system breaks down the digestible ones into sugar, which enters the blood.
- As blood sugar levels rise, the pancreas produces insulin, a hormone that prompts cells to absorb blood sugar for energy or storage.
- As cells absorb blood sugar, levels in the bloodstream begin to fall. When this happens, the pancreas start making glucagon, a hormone that signals the liver to start releasing stored sugar.
- This interplay of insulin and glucagon ensure that cells throughout the body, and especially in the brain, have a steady supply of blood sugar.
- The abuse of Carbohydrate consumption is important in the development of type 2 diabetes, which occurs when the body can't make enough insulin or can't properly use the insulin it makes.

- Type 2 diabetes usually develops gradually over a number of years, beginning when muscle and other cells stop responding to insulin. This condition, known as insulin resistance, causes blood sugar and insulin levels to stay high long after eating. Over time, the heavy demands made on the insulin-making cells wears them out, and insulin production eventually stops.
- http://www.hsph.harvard.edu/nutritionsource/carbohydrates/carbohydrates-and-blood-sugar/ (School of Public Health)

Diabetes Statistics:

- **Prevalence**: In 2012, 29.1 million Americans, or 9.3% of the population, had diabetes.
    - Approximately 1.25 million American children and adults have type 1 diabetes.

- **Undiagnosed**: Of the 29.1 million, 21.0 million were diagnosed, and 8.1 million were undiagnosed.

- **Prevalence in seniors**: The percentage of Americans age 65 and older remains high, at 25.9%, or 11.8 million seniors (diagnosed and undiagnosed).

- **New Cases**: The incidence of diabetes in 2012 was 1.7 million new diagnoses/year; in 2010 it was 1.9 million.

- **Prediabetes**: In 2012, 86 million Americans age 20 and older had prediabetes; this is up from 79 million in 2010.

- **Deaths**: Diabetes remains the 7th leading cause of death in the United States in 2010, with 69,071 death certificates listing it as the underlying cause of death, and a total of 234,051 death certificates listing diabetes as an underlying or contributing cause of death.

Breakdown by Ethnicity regarding Diabetes

- 7.6% of non-Hispanic whites
- 9.0% of Asian Americans
- 12.8% of Hispanics
- 13.2% of non-Hispanic blacks
- 15.9% of American Indians/Alaskan Natives

Complications/Co-Morbid Conditions :

http://www.diabetes.org/diabetes-basics/statistics/#sthash.5PzDiYdn.dpuf

- **Hypoglycemia**:
- **Hypertension**:
- **Dyslipidemia**:
- **Cardio Vascular Death Rates**:
- **Heart Attack Rates**:
- **Stroke**:
- **Blindness and Eye Problems**:
- **Amputations**:

Cost of Diabetes:

$245 billion: Total costs of diagnosed diabetes in the United States in 2012,

$176 billion for direct medical costs

$69 billion in reduced productivity

How Does Addiction Impact the Brain?

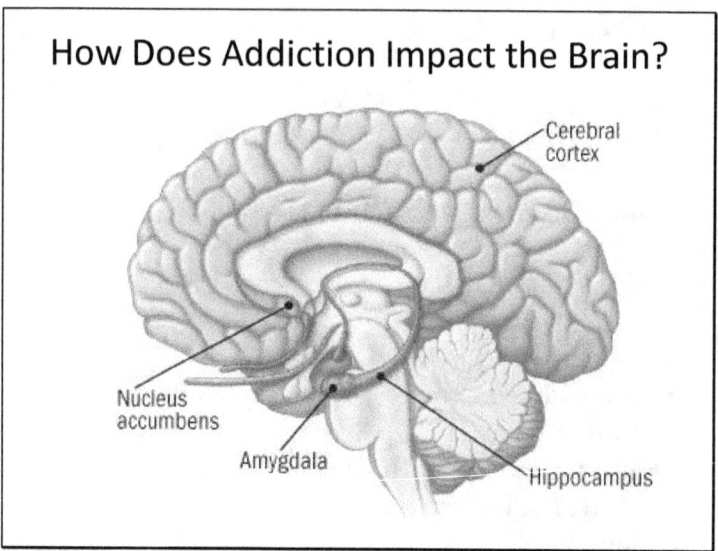

How Does Addiction Impact the Brain?

Cerebral cortex

Nucleus accumbens

Amygdala

Hippocampus

- In the brain, pleasure has a distinct signature: the release of the neurotransmitter *dopamine* in the **nucleus accumbens**, a cluster of nerve cells lying underneath the cerebral cortex (see illustration).
- *Dopamine* release in the **nucleus accumbens** is so consistently tied with pleasure that neuroscientists refer to the region as the brain's pleasure center. All drugs of abuse, from nicotine to heroin, cause a particularly powerful surge of **dopamine** in the **nucleus accumbens.**
- The likelihood that the use of a drug or participation in a rewarding activity will lead to addiction is directly linked to the speed with which it promotes *dopamine* release, the intensity of that release, and the reliability of that release. Addictive drugs provide a shortcut to the brain's reward system by flooding the **nucleus accumbens** with **dopamine**. The hippocampus lays down memories of this rapid sense of satisfaction, and the amygdala creates a conditioned response to certain stimuli. **Dopamine** not only contributes to the experience of pleasure, but also plays a role in learning and memory. According to the

current theory about addiction, **dopamine** interacts with another neurotransmitter, **glutamate**, to take over the brain's system of reward-related learning.

- This system has an important role in sustaining life because it links activities needed for **human survival** (such as eating and sex) with pleasure and reward. The reward circuit in the brain includes areas involved with motivation and memory as well as with pleasure. Addictive substances and behaviors stimulate the same circuit—and then overload it. Repeated exposure to an addictive substance or behavior causes nerve cells in the **nucleus accumbens** and the **prefrontal cortex** (the area of the brain involved in planning and executing tasks) to communicate in a way that couples liking something with wanting it, in turn driving us to go after it.

What is the Relationship between Tolerance and Addiction?

- In nature, rewards usually come only with time and effort. Addictive drugs and behaviors provide a shortcut, flooding the brain with **dopamine** and other **neurotransmitters**. Our brains do not have an easy way to withstand the onslaught. Addictive drugs, for example, can release **two to 10 times** the amount of **dopamine** that natural rewards do, and they do it more quickly and more reliably. In a person who becomes addicted, brain receptors become overwhelmed. The brain responds by producing **less dopamine** or eliminating dopamine receptors—. As a result of these adaptations, **dopamine** has less impact on the brain's reward center. People who develop an addiction typically find that, in time, the desired substance no longer gives them as much pleasure. They have to take more of it to obtain the same **dopamine "high"** because their brains have adapted—an effect known as tolerance.

Neurochemicals and Neurotransmitters

https://faculty.washington.edu/chudler/chnt1.html

- There may be underlying metabolic issues that predisposes certain people to ETOH abuse. These bio chemical changes may trigger the irreversible loss of control for some.
- The human brain utilizes glucose (fuel/energy) and water (oxygen) to function (Naff 2014). Glucose comes from carbohydrate foods. Carbohydrates are made up of complex sugars (vegetables, grains, cereals) and simple sugars (fruits, juice, milk). http://www.webmd.com/diabetes/blood-glucose
- A depletion or abuse in any of these resources will result in
  a. Poor cognition
  b. Inattention
  c. Memory problems/loss
  d. Cell damage or cell death.
- **Amino acids**: Are the building block for many neurotransmitters. Three amino acids that work with neurotransmitters are trypophan, taurine and tyrosine.
  - **Trypophan**: dairy products, eggs, nuts, fish and turkey.
  - **Taurine**: is a mood stabilizer, has a calming effect. Comes from meats, eggs and fish.
  - **Tyrosine**: soy products, chicken, turkey, fish, nuts, milk, cheese.

Neurotransmitters

- Neurotransmitters (help transport information through nerves) and proteins. They consist of dopamine, serotonin, norepinephrine, epinephrine, histamine.
- **Dopamine:** gives the body a natural "high" when something good happens (sexual activity, exercise, achievements, etc). It is depleted by processed sugar, caffeine, alcohol, sleep deprivation, and some anti-depressants). The symptoms of low dopamine are

low energy, boredom, craving sugar, caffeine, poor concertation, low sex drive, anxiety and depression.

- **Serotonin:** helps maintain mood levels, regulate the gastral intestinal track. It is depleted by alcohol, caffeine, nicotine, poor sunlight, exposure to heavy metals and pesticides. If elevated it can result in manic, psychotic behavior. If depleted is can result in low moods, irritability, poor sleeping patterns, anxiety, obsessive compulsive thoughts. It is improved by exercise, folic acid and exposure to sunlight.
- **Norepinephrine:** it helps suppress neuro inflammation, regulated glucose release, and regulated the endocrine system. It is responsible for fight/flight response, attention response, decision making and goal directed behavior. When elevated it may play a role of schizophrenia. When depleted is will manifest a low energy, loss of interest, low motivation and sleep disturbance.. What depletes it is cocaine, amphetamines. What helps is exercise and L-Tyrosine (amino acid) supplements.
- **Epinephrine:** its depletions can result in low blood pressure, excessive salt through kidneys, weight loss and chronic fatigue. What helps is sea salt and exercise.
- **Histamine:** it maintains vigilance and alertness. Elevated levels found in people suffering from schizophrenia. It is naturally found in meats and hard cheeses.

Food Warnings

Refined Sugars: reduce food nutrients and aggravates food intolerances.

Food Dyes: contribute to AHDA behaviors and allergies in children,

https://faculty.washington.edu/chudler/chnt1.html

Minerals and Vitamins that Support Mental Health

- **Lithium Oro-tate**: helps stabilize moods, reduces anxiety.

- **Magnesium:** helps sleep disturbances with ADHD children.
- **Iodine:** supports moods by maintaining energy levels and motivation. Maintains thyroid functions. Attained through sea kelp tablets.
- **Acetylcholine (Ah-seh –til – koleen)**: helps attention, decision making, learning ability, brain plasticity, supports memory. Found in Vitamin B5, vegetables, meats, cashew and eggs.
- **Vitamin B6, B12**: maintains healthy moods. Helps ADHD children.
- **Folic Acid:** helps the absorption of serotonin in the body.
- **Omega Fish Oils:** Helps with depression, supports brain activity, lower HDL cholesterol, keeps blood vessels clear, and improves oxygen flow to the brain.
  www.mdheal.org , www.mindingourbodies.ca , www.moodtracker.com , www.understandingaltmedicine.com, www.familydoctor.org, www.nutritionj.com, www.minddisorfers.com

The Psychological Impact of Addiction

- The **pleasure** associated with an addictive drug or behavior subsides—and yet the memory of the desired effect and the need to recreate it (the wanting) persists. The **hippocampus** and the **amygdala** store information about environmental cues associated with the desired substance, so that it can be located again. These **memories** help create a conditioned response—**intense craving**.
http://www.helpguide.org/harvard/addiction_hijacks_brain.htm

Social Behavioral Impact of Addictions

- Whenever the person encounters those **environmental cues**. A person addicted to heroin may be in danger of relapse when he sees a hypodermic needle, for example, while another person might start to drink again after **seeing** a bottle of whiskey. Conditioned learning helps explain why people who develop an addiction risk relapse even after years of abstinence. *http://www.helpguide.org/harvard/addiction_hijacks_brain.htm*

Treatment Goals

- Motive that the client to accept the need for help.
- Receive detox treatment for the medical problems related to withdrawal symptoms.
- Develop new behaviors that will prevent them from relapsing into the addictive cycle.
- Help them develop coping skills to rebuild relationships damaged by the addictive behaviors.
- Encourage them to utilize family counseling.
- Assist them in developing resources that will assist in the recovery process. Help the family members to recognize co-dependency issues or family behaviors that may facilitate the addictions. Plug the client into support groups like A.A support groups (Asquith,2010).

Contemporary Solutions Utilized to Manage Addictions

Medical Intervention: Utilization of medical detoxification regime (in patient medical facility) that may be a few days until the patient is stabilized. Assign a psychiatrics or internal medicine physician to administer medication management with nursing care. Then given a social worker or case manager to plan after care treatment.

Psychological/ Behavioral Health Intervention: They are assigned a mental health counselor or psychologist for one on one treatment. Work on the behavioral and emotional factors that contribute to the compulsive addictive behavior. These sessions can be three to eight meetings. It also depends the philosophical orientation of the therapist. Some relationships may continue for a few years.

Social workers and Case Managers: Due to the severity of the addictive process on their interpersonal relationships. They will need considerable assistance in basic living sustenance. May become indigent and homeless or have dependent children who need care and assistance. Many are unemployed, disabled or considered un employable due to criminal backgrounds. They are in need of considerable social assistance.

Group Therapy: Support groups ran by professional clinicians with the same goals as individual counseling but with a greater focus on psychological educational materials.

Community of Faith: A community organized around a common belief, creed, philosophical mindset or covenant. They provide counseling or pastoral care services to members of their particular community.

Self-Help Groups: These groups are directed by nonprofessionals and peers. Typically the leaders are folks who have recovered or in the process of recovering from addictive disorders. Examples of these groups are Celebrate Recovery and 12- Step groups.

Faith Community Based Prevention

- Offer parent education that focuses on nurturing the self-esteem and the sense of responsibility within children and youth. Offer topics that focus on addiction prevention and self-defeating behaviors.
- Offer ETOH education and counseling services that will help develop construct social attitudes and controls regarding ETOH abuse.

- Focus on parents that struggle with addiction. That will help their children avoid the same future pitfalls.

Views on Spirituality

- As the brain processes sensory experiences, we naturally look for patterns, and then seek out **meaning in those patterns**. And the phenomenon known as "cognitive dissonance" shows that once we believe in something, we will try to explain away anything that conflicts with it. http://www.psychologytoday.com/basics/spirituality
- The state or quality of being dedicated to God, religion, or spiritual things or **values**, in contrasted with material or temporal ones. http://dictionary.reference.com/browse/spirituality
- Spirituality refers to any religious or ethical value that is made concrete as an attitude or spirit from which one's actions flow.
- Paul Evdokimov: "the life of man facing his God, participating in the life of God; the spirit of man listening for the Spirit of God.")
- The spiritual life is a supernatural life.
- Belief in a universal being.
- Communicating with this being through the act of prayer, meditation or contemplation.
- It is a sense of being connected with others.
- Positive experience of a direct relationship with a transcendent being.
- A sense of wholeness.
- A sense of unity with life.
- A higher plane of consciousness
- A spirituality that binds all people together.
- Sense of strong emotional ties with others.
- Universality – sense of unity with life.

Gallop Poll 2007, Piedmont 1999, Piedmont 2010
Asire-SF, Piedmont 2010

What are Sacred Moments

- Report the feelings of transcendence, ultimacy, boundlessness, interconnectedness and spiritual emotion.
- Experiences set apart from normal everyday reality.
- Extends beyond the limited self.
- Initiates new growth, insights motivation and satisfaction, meaningfulness and ultimate well-being.
- Create fundamental transformations in behavior.
- Created from a synergy between client and counselor.

www.sciencedaily.com/releases/2015/01/150105170243.htm

The Role of the Community of Faith

There are a couple of things the community of faith can do regarding ETOH abuse with their congregations.

- Through sermons and teachings, the topic of addiction can be addressed. An atmosphere of openness should be fostered that will encourage people to seek help.
- Pastoral care and counseling services should be offered to assist the addict and the family members effected within the congregation. The church can be a meeting place for support groups that address addictions for both the client and family members (p178).
- The community of faith leader can be a significant support for the addict their family during this time of crisis (Asquith, 2010)

Bill Wilson's Sacred Moment

Bill was admitted to a New York Hospital on his 39th birthday. He was desperate to change his life that was dominated by alcoholism. So he pleaded with God stating that he would do anything at all to change. He then described the next experience "suddenly, my room blazed with an indescribably bright white light…then seen with his mind eye a mountain. Upon the summit a great wind blew. It was a spirit, a great clean strength that blew right through me. Then came a blazing thought "You are free". From that moment he never doubted the existence of God and never took another drink of alcohol.

The Oxford Group

- Started by Dr. Frank Buchman a Swiss Lutheran Priest in 1908 and supported by Rev. Cosmo Land the Anglican Bishop of Canterbury in England.
- The groups started on the Oxford University (England) campus among the students and staff from 1930 to 1937 and group among the community of faith involving 1,000 clergy, 5000 lay people and 12 bishops
- Believed the roots of all personal problems were grounded in fear and selfishness. That the solution or remedy is the act of surrender to God. This is an act of humility.
- Spoke about the Four Absolutes: Absolute honesty, absolute purity, absolute unselfishness and absolute love.

The Spiritual Practice:
- Sharing of our sins and temptations with others.
- Surrender our past life, present and future into God's keeping.
- Restitution to all those who have wronged directly or indirectly.
- Listening for God's guidance and carrying it out.

The Five C's and Five Procedures:
- Confidence: the people will have assurance that you will honor the confidentiality of others
- Confession: Ability to honest about the real state of your life
- Conversion: The free will decision to turn ones life over to God.
- Continuance: Work towards sharing the life-changing journey with others who suffer.
  En.Wikipedia.org/Oxford_Group.

The 12-Step Program History

- The Oxford Group "laid particular emphasis on spiritual principles that we needed.
- The <u>12 step program</u> itself is over seventy years old.
- The <u>12 steps</u> followed the creation of <u>A.A.</u> by a few years, and they did not come into being all at once; rather, they developed somewhat organically before coming together in a very short period of time while co-founder <u>Bill Wilson</u> was writing what would become the Big Book in 1938.
- He reached the realization that a book was not enough, that they needed a specific <u>program</u> for recovery. A number of the steps had already existed though mostly by word-of-mouth; Wilson's epiphany was to put what existed under a single banner and add to them what might have been missing.
- Those original <u>12 steps</u> featured the use of God on several occasions, which Wilson reduced down to the minimum. The famous qualifier "as we understood Him" was not added until later. Beyond that, according to Wilson, the 12 steps "stand today almost exactly as they were first written."
- Since then those 12 steps have been adopted by numerous organizations to deal with everything from narcotics abuse to emotional disorders and more.
  http://www.12step.com/history.html

Step 1
We admit we are powerless over (addiction)—that our lives have become unmanageable.

[18] For I know that nothing good dwells in me, that is, in my flesh; for the willing is present in me, but the doing of the good *is* not. [19] For the good that I want, I do not do, but I practice the very evil that I do not want. [20] But if I am doing the very thing I do not want, I am no longer the one doing it, but sin which dwells in me. [21] I find then the [a]principle that evil is present in me, the one who wants to do good.[22] For I joyfully concur with the law of God [b]in the inner man, [23] but I see a different law in [c]the members of my body, waging war against the law of my mind and making me

a prisoner [d]of the law of sin which is in my members. (Romans 7:18-23) (NASB)

Reflection: The need for confession regarding the addiction and the impact it has made on daily life.
- Coming to grips with reality of our lives and ourselves.
- Heartfelt admission of self-defeating and self-destructive behavior.
- The admission of our need to surrender the control of our addictive selves to a Power greater than ourselves. Pg 6.

The 12 Steps: A Spiritual Journey. Recovery Publication, San Diago CA. 1988

Questions to ask: (p 9 -22)
- Are their excessive feelings over which I am powerless?
- Are their behaviors which I am powerless?
- Are there people over whom I feel powerless?

A Hunger for Healing, J. Keith Miller, HarperSanFrancisco. 1991.

Step 2
We come to believe that a Power greater than ourselves can restore us to sanity.

Scripture: Matthew 11:28-30 (NASB) **28** "Come to Me, all [a]who are weary and heavy-laden, and I will give you rest. **29** Take My yoke upon you and learn from Me, for I am gentle and humble in heart, and you will find rest for your souls. **30** For My yoke is [b]easy and My burden is light."

Reflection: This is an act of humility. The sufferer understands that only a power greater than himself and the addiction can restore his mind and heart.
- Involves an active effort to place one trust in God or Higher Power.
- Start to believe that a Power greater than ourselves will restore us to sanity and wellbeing. P.14.

The 12 Steps: A Spiritual Journey. Recovery Publication, San Diago CA. 1988

Questions to Ask: (28 -33)
- What areas do you experience reoccurring fears?
- To who do you experience repeated resentment?
- What are your repeated self-defeating behaviors?
- Think of an instance when you did something "crazy" that resulted in harm to you or another?
- Think of a time when you refused to get help when you knew you really needed it?

A Hunger for Healing, J. Keith Miller, HarperSanFrancisco. 1991.

Step 3
We make a decision to turn our will and our lives over to the care of God as we understand Him.

Scripture: Matthew 4:18 -23 (NASB): **"Now as Jesus was walking by the Sea of Galilee, He saw two brothers, Simon who was called Peter, and Andrew his brother, casting a net into the sea; for they were fishermen. [19] And He *said to them, "[a]Follow Me, and I will make you fishers of men."[20] Immediately they left their nets and followed Him. [21] Going on from there He saw two other brothers, [b]James the *son* of Zebedee, and [c]John his brother, in the boat with Zebedee their father, mending their nets; and He called them. [22] Immediately they left the boat and their father, and followed Him. [23] Jesus was going throughout all Galilee, teaching in their synagogues and proclaiming the [d]gospel of the kingdom, and healing every kind of disease and every kind of sickness among the people."**

Reflection: *The suffering makes a conscious free willed choice to turn his life over to God and the church.*

Reflection on Step 3
- Start to acknowledge the need for God (Higher Power) in our lives
- Be prepare to surrender ourselves to Him. P.27

The 12 Steps: A Spiritual Journey. Recovery Publication, San Diago CA. 1988

Questions to ask:
- Were you raised with "do it by yourself" or "take care of yourself" messages?
- What does the thought of surrendering complete control to "Another" feel like? What does this feel like?
- What messages regarding boundaries did you hear from your parents growing up?
- What are reason why you cannot trust God?
- Were you able to trust your parents growing up?

A Hunger for Healing, J. Keith Miller, HarperSanFrancisco. 1991.

Step 4: We make a searching and fearless moral inventory of ourselves.

Luke 12: 1-3 (NASB): "Under these circumstances, after [a]so many thousands of [b]people had gathered together that they were stepping on one another, He began saying to His disciples first of all, "Beware of the leaven of the Pharisees, which is hypocrisy. [2] But there is nothing covered up that will not be revealed, and hidden that will not be known. [3] Accordingly, whatever you have said in the dark will be heard in the light, and what you have[c]whispered in the inner rooms will be proclaimed upon the housetops."

Guidelines for Step 4:

The 12 Steps: A Spiritual Journey. Recovery Publication, San Diago CA. 1988 (p 51 to
- Develop a deeper self-knowledge leading to self-acceptance and and self-love.
- Facing the truth about our behavior.
- Identifying behavior patterns and surrendering the them.
- Finding a sponsor and attending meetings.

Reflection: The sufferer starts a personal scrutiny of all (from the beginning) the negative things he has done as a result of the addictive lifestyle chosen.

Coming face to face with the denial regarding the self-defeating, self destructive behaviors.

Willingness to deal with the following behaviors:

Resentment: From swollen instincts, clashing with others, violent feelings and childhood memories.

- With whom?
- What was the cause?
- How did this affect my life?
- What did you do in response?

Fears: Happens when self-reliance fails, or when our faith fails or when someone we trust let us down.

- Identify the fear
- What was the cause?
- How did it affect me?

Swollen Instincts: Think specifically of the times when self-centeredness caused you harm. Focus on specific behaviors and attitudes.

- **Sexual Instincts:** Think of each relationship and behaviors.
- **Financial Security:** what are your insecurities regarding money. What are your spending habits?
- **Emotional Security:** Times when you were over dependent and/or excessively controlling over someone else due to insecurity.
- **Social Instincts:** what are your thoughts regarding status among your peers , group or organizational situations? Do you the center of attention? Or the smartest person in the room? Are you a wall flower? Do you disappear in the group?

A Hunger for Healing, J. Keith Miller, HarperSanFrancisco. 1991. (p72)

Step 5: We admit to God, to ourselves, and to another human being the exact nature of our wrongs.

Scripture: James 5:16 NASB): *"[16] Therefore, confess your sins to one another, and pray for one another so that you may be healed. The effective [a]prayer of a righteous man can accomplish much."*

Reflection: This is an act of confession. This involves humility and the willingness to confess the extent of harm done to the very people injured by the addicted lifestyle.

- Acknowledging and discarding old survival skills.
- Transitioning to new and healthier lifestyle.
- Do a thorough and honest personal inventory of all behaviors (thoughts, words and deeds).
- Willing to both face the facts and move forward. p70

The 12 Steps: A Spiritual Journey. Recovery Publication, San Diago CA. 1988

The Three Phases:

- Choose someone to whom you can fully admit the exact nature of you self-defeating and self-destructive lifestyle.
- Meet with that person and discuss what you have learned in Step 4.
- Be willing to receive feedback from that person regarding what you have shared.

Reflection of the Three Phases:

- What were your feeling during your meeting with your 5th Step person?
- Did you discover something new about yourself from this experience?
- What are your feelings now that you have completed your 5th step?

- *A Hunger for Healing, J. Keith Miller, HarperSanFrancisco. 1991. (p72)*

Step 6: We are entirely ready to have God remove all these defects of character.

Scripture: *(Romans 6: 8 – 11)* NASB⁺ *"⁵ For if we have become [a]united with Him in the likeness of His death, certainly we shall also be [b]in the likeness of His resurrection, ⁶ knowing this, that our old[c]self was crucified with Him, in order that our body of sin might be [d]done away with, so that we would no longer be **slaves** to sin; ⁷ for he who has died is [e]freed from sin. ⁸ Now if we have died with Christ, we believe that we shall also live with Him,⁹ knowing that Christ, having been raised from the dead, [f]is never to die again; death no longer is master over Him. ¹⁰ For the death that He died, He died to sin once for all; but the life that He lives, He lives to God. ¹¹ Even so consider yourselves to be dead to sin, but alive to God in Christ Jesus.*

Reflection:
- This is an act of humility, healing and consecration. The sufferer is willing to allow God and the church to do whatever it takes to bring healing to the person's mind, body and soul.
- Have a sincere desire and change in behavior and lifestyle.
- Be willing to call upon Higher power for help
- Fully recognizing ones life condition. Honest determination to eliminate self defeating behaviors.
- In what way did you try to fix yourself but failed?
- Have you identified character defeats that will require God to heal?
- Are there character defeats you have struggles letting go of?
- Are you engaging in religious behaviors that are self-defeating?
- Are there times when have attempted to "fix" or manipulate others with your own power?

A Hunger for Healing, J. Keith Miller, HarperSanFrancisco. 1991. (p87)

Step 7: We humbly ask Him to remove our shortcomings.

Scripture: *"(1 Peter 5:6-11)NASB: "⁶ Therefore humble yourselves under the mighty hand of God, that He may exalt you at the proper time, ⁷ casting all your anxiety on Him, because He cares for you. ⁸ Be of sober spirit, be on the alert. Your adversary, the devil, prowls around like a roaring lion, seeking someone to devour. ⁹ [d] But resist him, firm in your faith, knowing that the same experiences of suffering are being accomplished by your [e] brethren who are in the world. ¹⁰ After you have suffered for a little while, the God of all grace, who called you to His eternal glory in Christ, will Himself perfect, confirm, strengthen and establish you. ¹¹ To Him be dominion forever and ever. Amen"*

Reflection: This is an act of humility and confession. Again the sufferer is asking God to bring healing and restoration to his damaged mind, body and soul.

- Acknowledging the benefits given us in life.
- Grateful for God's presences.
- Reviewing the success of letting go of self defeating behavior. p90
- Reflect on the term Humility. What does it mean?
- Think of specific times when you acted out of pride.
- Think of positive behaviors that will replace identified self-defeating behaviors.
- Record when you observe yourself replacing the negative behavers with positive ones.

A Hunger for Healing, J. Keith Miller, HarperSanFrancisco. 1991. (p87)

Step 8

We make a list of all persons we have harmed, and become willing to make amends to them all.

Scripture: Luke 19:8-10 (NASB) : [8] Zaccheus stopped and said to the Lord, "Behold, Lord, half of my possessions I [a]will give to the poor, and if I have defrauded anyone of anything, I [b]will give back four times as much." [9] And Jesus said to him, "Today salvation has come to this house, because he, too, is a son of Abraham. [10] For the Son of Man has come to seek and to save that which was lost."

Reflection: This is an act of humility, confession, restitution and reconciliation. The sufferer makes a thorough list and inventory of every person they have harmed due to the addiction. They are also willing to make amends to those people however possible.

Reflection on Step 8

- Begin the process if healing damaged relationships by making amends for past behaviors.
- Continued working on letting go of resentments, guilt, shame, low self-esteem and past self-defeating behaviors.
- Work on developing newly acquired relational skills.
- Continue to do self-reflection on material, moral and spiritual wrongs done to self and others. p102

The 12 Steps: A Spiritual Journey. Recovery Publication, San Diago CA. 1988

- Make a list of all the people harmed by my behaviors. Identify what happened and the resulting consequences.
- What feelings come up for you as you think about the behaviors and consequences?
- Make a list of all the people who harmed you, what they did, the consequence and how you fell about it today.

- Practice writing a statement of forgiveness towards each person who wronged you.
- Write a statement of readiness to make amends to each person you have harmed.

A Hunger for Healing, J. Keith Miller, HarperSanFrancisco. 1991. (p110)

Step 9: We make direct amends to such people wherever possible, except when to do so would injure them or others.

Scripture: Matthew 5:23 (NASB) [23] "Therefore if you are presenting your [a]offering at the altar, and there remember that your brother has something against you,"

Refection: This is an act of humility and reconciliation. There is a conscious and humbled effort to make amends to every person injured or harmed by the addicted behavior.

- Review the list in Step 8 and develop a concrete action plan to make each amend.
- The goal is to make the amends as complete as possible.
- Some amends can take effect by simply changing ones behavior towards others.
- If you are unable to reconcile with the injured party an work of Charity to the needy will suffice. p112

The 12 Steps: A Spiritual Journey. Recovery Publication, San Diago CA. 1988

- Make a physical list of every person you would like to seek amends. Document the date, method, restitution needed and feelings experienced.
- Make a list of the people you are not willing to make amends and the reason why.

A Hunger for Healing, J. Keith Miller, HarperSanFrancisco. 1991. (p122)

Step 10: We continue to take personal inventory and when we are wrong promptly admitted it.

Step 10

Scripture: Philippians 2:12-13 (NASB): [12] So then, my beloved, just as you have always obeyed, not as in my presence only, but now much more in my absence, work out your salvation with fear and trembling;[13] for it is God who is at work in you, both to will and to work for *His* good pleasure.

Reflection: This involves humility. The suffer takes personal examination of all thoughts, words and actions is a daily.
- Develop a capacity for self-appraisal.
- Develop the disciple of a work/effort and natural reward experience This takes cultivating patients and self control.
- Focus on maintaining inventories:
- Daily inventory: At the end of the day do a self-evaluation.
- Spot-Check inventory: few times a day (like checking your pulse)
- Long –Term Periodic Inventory: The occurs at a retreat, workshop, respite, contemplative or meditative exercise. P.122

The 12 Steps: A Spiritual Journey. Recovery Publication, San Diago CA. 1988

Daily Inventory Example:
- Describe the incident
- What/whom are you powerless over?
- What self-defeating thoughts/behaviors occurred from which you need God's help?
- Write out your decision to turn that situation over to God.
- If you failed, how will you make amends?
- Work on a Gratitude list once a month or quarter.
- Review Step 3 : **We make a decision to turn our will and our lives over to the care of God as we understand Him.**
- Do I periodic (monthly, quarterly) list of people you may have harmed and the restitution needed to make amends.

A Hunger for Healing, J. Keith Miller, HarperSanFrancisco. 1991. (p122)

Step 11

We seek through prayer and <u>meditation</u> to improve our conscious contact with God as we understand Him, praying only for knowledge of His Will for us and the power to carry that out.

Scripture: 1 Peter 4:1-8 (NASB) "Therefore, since Christ has [a]suffered in the flesh, arm yourselves also with the same purpose, because he who has [b]suffered in the flesh has ceased from sin, ² so as to live the rest of the time in the flesh no longer for the lusts of men, but for the will of God. ³ For the time already past is sufficient *for you* to have carried out the desire of the Gentiles, [c]having pursued a course of sensuality, lusts, drunkenness, carousing, drinking parties and [d]abominable idolatries. ⁴ In *all* this, they are surprised that you do not run with *them* into the same excesses of dissipation, and they malign *you*; ⁵ but they will give account to Him who is ready to judge the living and the dead. ⁶ For the gospel has for this purpose been [e]preached even to those who are dead, that though they are judged in the flesh as men, they may live in the spirit according to *the will of* God. ⁷ The end of all things [f]is near; therefore, be of sound judgment and sober *spirit* for the purpose of [g]prayer. ⁸ Above all, keep fervent in your love for one another, because love covers a multitude of sins."

Reflection: This is an act of humility and consecration. The sufferer engages in active spiritual and religious exercises that will strengthen their personal relationship with God and with other people.

Reflection of Step 11

- Asking for God's will for our lives and the strength to fulfill that purpose.
- The strength to set aside self serving behaviors and motives
- Experience a sense of serenity and peace regarding this new journey of recovery and health. p132. The 12 Steps: A

Spiritual Journey. Recovery Publication, San Diago CA.
1988

- Finding time daily for prayer and meditation. Are there difficulties doing this?
- Are you "playing God" doing this time of prayer and meditation?
- Are you experiencing nudges or insights during this time? Why or why not? Write down what you are perceiving during these times.
- Did you implement the nudges? Why or why not?
- Think about practice visualization during this time. What do you see?

A Hunger for Healing, J. Keith Miller, HarperSanFrancisco. 1991. (p122)

Step 12

Having had a spiritual awakening as the result of these steps, we try to carry this message to alcoholics, and to practice these <u>principles</u> in all our affairs.

Scriptures: Galatians 6:1-2 (NASB) "Brethren, even if [a]anyone is caught in any trespass, you who are spiritual, restore such a one in a spirit of gentleness; *each one* looking to yourself, so that you too will not be tempted. [2] Bear one another's burdens, and thereby fulfill the law of Christ."

Reflection: This is an act of evangelism and mercy. The sufferer actively **looks for** opportunities to share his spiritual experiences with others who are suffering. He is also willing to bring people physically to the 12 step meeting whenever possible.
<u>http://12step.org/bibl/step-12-scriptures.html</u>

Reflection of Step 12

- The call to share the 12 Step message to others.
- Be willing to share ones own experience of prayer and meditation.
- Be willing to share the journey of working through the steps with others struggling with addiction.
- Telling your personal story to others is a humbling step that takes courage. p 140
- Write out your spiritual awakening.
    - What were you like during your addiction?
    - What was the crisis that brought you to this spiritual awakening?
    - What is now different about your life?
    - What are your realizations? Your new hopes? Hope do you now perceive reality? Have you found meaning through your suffering?

APPENDIX

Case Study 1:

April a single mother with a strong faith background. She came into counseling regarding her angry teenage son. His biological father left the family due to drug addiction and marital infidelity when the boy was two years old. His father had little contact with his son. As a teenager, the boy was sneaking out of the house to attend parties and abuse drugs. This resulted in him being expelled from faith based private school due to his anger against authority figures and other students. He was also accused of sexually abusing a fellow female student. How would you help this mother and her son?

Case Study 2:

Michelle a 21 year woman was in the hospital for a drug overdose. She got involved with a drug group and gang as a teenager and would exchange sex for drugs. Her addiction became stronger and she engaged in riskier sexual behavior. Her sexual behavior increased her guilt until she finally overdosed. She was raised in a religious family. How would you counsel her?

Case Study 3:

Jennifer a 19 year old female was hospitalized due to a multiple suicide attempts. She swallowed a large amount of prescription medications and narcotics. She had a history of drug abuse and was involved in a long term homosexual relationship that ended suddenly. Her family members are actively involved in the Gay community. She reported multiple prior hospitalizations for drug abuse. As a result of her failed relationship she attempted suicide. She asked for prayer and spiritual counseling. How would you help her?

Case Study 4:

Jerry was in his late 60's. He was a Vietnam Veteran who served three tours in the Special Forces as a Captain. After returning state side, he developed a drug and alcohol addiction and struggled with the memories of what he had seen and done in the military. He became a successful aeronautical engineer and college professor earning a PH.D. He had three failed marriages due to serial infidelities. He had three children he had not seen in years. He experienced a medical episode that brought him to the intensive care unit. This was life threatening. He asked for prayer support. How would you counsel him?

Case Study 5:

Cathy, a 34 - year old woman, was admitted to the hospital for suicide attempt by drug overdose. She stated she was raped by her biological father from the age of 3. At 13 years old she became pregnant and lost her first baby. Her father was a very violent man and was an active member of a hate group during childhood. As a teenager she abused drugs and became sexually involved with multiple violent men. Her current boyfriend threatened to kill her and her three children. She asked for prayer support. How would you offer her spiritual care?

Case Study 6:

Jim came to counseling under duress after separating from his wife and leaving pastoral ministry. He reported struggling with pornography and infidelity during his marriage. He grew up in a family with a generational history of alcoholism and infidelity. The message he got was that "boys will be boys". That history has ruined his marriage and ministry. How would you help him? How would you his spiritual needs?

Case Study # 7:

Michael was a famous and successful Christian author. He is married with four kids. However he had a secret sexual addiction. He viewed pornography and would inappropriately touch women in public. He was eventually caught and was ordered to enter counseling. How would you counsel him?

Holy Scripture and Addictions

- 1 Peter 5:8: *"Be sober-minded; be watchful. Your adversary the* **devil** *prowls around like a roaring lion, seeking someone to* **devour."**

- John 8:34: *"Very truly I tell you, everyone who sins is a* **slave** *to sin"*

- Matthew 6:13: *"And lead us not into temptation, but deliver us from* **evil.** *"*

- Colossians 3:5: "Put to death therefore what is earthly in you: sexual immorality, impurity, passion, **evil** desire, and covetousness, which is idolatry."

- James 4:7: "Submit yourselves therefore to God. Resist the **devil,** and he will flee from you."

1 John 3:8: **"**Whoever makes a practice of sinning is of the **devil,** for the **devil** has been sinning from the beginning. The reason the Son of God appeared was to destroy the works of the **devil.**"

Roman Catholic Sacraments a Source of Healing for the Person Struggling with Addiction:

What is the Definition Evil? Evil, in a large sense, may be described as the sum of the opposition, which experience shows to exist in the universe, to the desires and needs of individuals; whence arises, among human beings at least, the sufferings in which life abounds.

What is the Definition of Moral Evil? *Moral* evils are understood to be the deviation of human volition from the prescriptions of the moral order and the action which results from that deviation. The solution for men to find freedom from evil is the gracious application of God's grace.

What is the Definition of Grace?

1. Grace (*gratia, Charis*), in general, is a supernatural gift of God to intellectual creatures (men, angels) for their eternal salvation.
2. Eternal salvation itself consists in heavenly bliss resulting from the intuitive knowledge of the Triune God.
3. Christian grace is a fundamental idea of the <u>Christian religion</u>, the pillar on which, by a special ordination of God, the majestic edifice of Christianity rests in its entirety. Among the three fundamental ideas — sin, redemption, and grace — grace plays the part of the means, indispensable and Divinely ordained, to effect the redemption from sin through Christ and to lead men to their eternal destiny in heaven.
http://www.newadvent.org/cathen/06701a.htm

What Does Holy Scripture say about Suffering?

Scriptural Reference to Suffering:

1. *"Indeed I count everything as loss because of the surpassing worth of knowing Christ Jesus my Lord. For his sake I have suffered the loss of all things, and count them as refuse, in order that I may gain Christ and be found in him, not having a righteousness of my own, based on law, but that which is through faith in Christ, the righteousness from God depends on faith; that I may know him and the power of his resurrection, and may share his **suffering**, becoming like him in his death, that if possible I may attain the resurrection from the dead"* (Philippians 3:8-11)

2. *"For I know that through your prayers and the help of the Spirit of Jesus Christ this will turn out for my **deliverance,** as it is my eager expectation and hope that I shall not be at all ashamed, but that with full courage now as always Christ will be honored in my body, whether by life or by death. For to me to live is Christ and to die is gain"* (Philippians 1:19-21).

3.   *'My grace is sufficient for you, for my power is made perfect in* **weakness**.*'...For the sake of Christ, then, I am content with* **weaknesses, insults, hardships, persecutions, and calamities**; *for when I am weak then I am strong" (2 Corinthians 12:7-10).*

Definition of Sacraments:

1. An outward sign of inward grace,
    a sacred and mysterious sign or ceremony, ordained by Christ, by which grace is conveyed to our souls for our sanctification. The principal reason for a sacramental system is found in man.
2.   It is the nature of man, writes St. Thomas (III:61:1), to be led by things corporeal and sense-perceptible to things spiritual and intelligible; now Divine Providence provides for everything in accordance with its nature; therefore it is fitting that Divine Wisdom should provide means of salvation for men in the form of certain corporeal and sensible signs which are called sacraments.

3. The Sacrament is the cause and agent of that grace in the souls of men. A sacrosanct sign producing grace, Sacrament, in its broadest acceptation, may be defined as an external sign of something sacred. The sign of a sacred thing in so far as it sanctifies men. In every sacrament three things are necessary: the outward sign; the inward grace; Divine institution. http://www.newadvent.org/cathen/13295a.htm.

Personal Reflection: From my experience with inpatient psychiatric patients, they will ask for prayer or an external intervention to help them with the addiction and the addictive lifestyle surrounding their drug of choice.

1. **Sacrament of Baptism as Cure for the Addicted Soul.**

    a. Holy Baptism holds the first place among the sacraments, because it is the door of the spiritual life; for by it we are made members of Christ and incorporated with the Church.

    b. And since through the first man death entered into all, unless we be born again of water and the Holy Ghost, we cannot enter into the kingdom of Heaven, as Truth Himself has told us.
        http://www.newadvent.org/cathen/02258b.htm

Scripture

(Acts 2:38): *"Be baptized every one of you in the name of Jesus Christ, for the remission of your sins; and you shall receive the Holy Ghost. For the promise is to you and to your children and to all that are far off, whomsoever the Lord our God shall call."*

(Acts 22:16): *"Be baptized, and wash away thy sins." St. Paul in the fifth chapter of his Epistle to the Ephesians beautifully represents the whole Church as being baptized and purified (5:25 sq.): "Christ loved the Church, and delivered Himself up for it: that he might sanctify it, cleansing it by the washing of water in the word of life: that he might present it to Himself a glorious Church, not having spot or wrinkle, or any such thing; but that it should be holy and without blemish.*

Reflection: The Baptismal promises exercises out evil from the sufferer's life and gives them the capacity to resist falling under the powerful influence of the addictive cycle. By reflecting on those promises daily, the sufferer can be reassured that he has the power and the strength to overcome the devastating effects of the addiction. It also brings into realization that addiction is an attack of evil.

2.   Sacrament of Confirmation as Cure for the Addicted Soul.

   a.   A sacrament in which the Holy Ghost is given to those
        already baptized in order to make them strong and
        perfect Christians and soldiers of Jesus Christ.

   b.   It has been variously designated: a making fast or
        endure; a perfecting or completing, as expressing its
        relation to baptism. With reference to its effect it is the
        "Sacrament of the Holy Ghost", the "Sacrament of the
        Seal". From the external rite it is known as the
        "imposition of hands", or as "anointing with chrism".
        http://www.newadvent.org/cathen/04215b.htm

Scripture: Acts of the Apostles (8:14-17) that after
the Samaritan converts had been baptized by Philip the
deacon, the Apostles "sent unto them Peter and John, who,
when they were come, prayed for them, that they might
receive the Holy Ghost; for he was not yet come upon any of
them, but they were only baptized in the name of theLord
Jesus; then they laid their hands upon them, and they
received the Holy Ghost".

Reflection: This sacrament provides a special anointing and
seal for the believer. They are empowered to fulfill God's
purpose for their lives and have the capacities to resist evil.
They are filled with the virtues and gifts of the Holy Spirit.
This enables them to live a righteous life and live out the
fruits of the Holy Spirits.

3.   Sacrament of the Eucharist as Cure for the Addicted Soul.

a. *Since Christ is present under the appearances of bread and wine in a sacramental way, the Blessed Eucharistis is a sacrament of the Church. Indeed, in the Eucharist the definition of a Christian sacrament as "an outward sign of an inward grace instituted by Christ" is verified.*

b. There are two Eucharistic elements, bread and wine, which constitute the remote matter of the Sacrament of the Altar, while the proximate matter can be none other than the Eucharistic appearances under which the Body and Blood of Christ are truly present http://www.newadvent.org/cathen/05584a.htm

Scripture:

Matthew 26:26-28: Now as they were eating, Jesus took bread, and blessed, and broke it, and gave it to the disciples and said, "Take, eat; this is my body." And he took a cup, and when he had given thanks he gave it to them, saying, "Drink of it, all of you; for this is my blood of the covenant, which is poured out for many for the forgiveness of sins.

Reflection: The Holy Eucharist literally brings the physical presence of Christ into the body of the sufferer and empowers the person to resist the powerful lure of the addiction. It also reminds the sufferer that Christ also suffered in the body and through Him we can endure the temptation and have hope for the resurrection.

4. **Sacrament of the Extreme Unction (Anointing of the Sick) as Cure for the Addicted Soul.**

    a. A sacrament of the New Law instituted by Christ to give spiritual aid and comfort and perfect spiritual health,

    b. It provides the remission of sins, and also, conditionally, to restore bodily health, to Christians who are seriously ill; it consists essentially in the unction by a priest of the

body of the sick person, accompanied by a
suitable form of words.
http://www.newadvent.org/cathen/05716a.htm

Scripture: *James 5:14-15 "Is any man sick among you?
Let him bring in the priests of the Church, and let
them pray over him, anointing him with oil in the name of
the Lord. And the prayer of faith shall save [sosei] the
sick man: and the Lord shall raise him up [egerei]: and if
he be in sins, they shall be forgiven him."*

Refection: Grace and mercy is conferred on those who
may suffer. If they have sin they will be forgiven. It is
also a time to exorcize away evil and torment. This
sacrament allows peace to enter the troubled mind, body
and soul.

5.   **Sacrament of Marriage as Cure for the Addicted Soul.**

The classical Scriptural text is the declaration of
the Apostle Paul who emphatically declares that the
relation between husband and wife should be as the
relation between Christ and His Church:
http://www.newadvent.org/cathen/09707a.htm

I would get a different version:
Scripture: *(Ephesians 5:22 sqq.), "Let women be subject
to their husbands, as to the Lord: because the husband is
the head of the wife, as Christ is the head of the Church.
He is the saviour of his body. Therefore as the Church is
subject to Christ, so also let the wives be to their
husbands in all things. Husbands, love your wives,
as Christ also loved the Church, and delivered Himself
up for it: that He might sanctify it, cleansing it by the
laver of water in the word of life; that He might present it
to Himself a glorious church not having spot or wrinkle
or any such thing; but that it should be holy, and without
blemish. So also ought men to love their wives as their*

own bodies. He that loveth his wife, loveth himself. For no man ever hated his own flesh; but nourisheth it and cherisheth it, as also Christ doth the Church: because we are members of His body, of His flesh, and of His bones." After this exhortation theApostle alludes to the Divine institution of marriage in the prophetical words proclaimed by God through Adam: "For this cause shall a man leave his father and mother and shall cleave to his wife, and they shall be two in one flesh." He then concludes with the significant words in which he characterizes Christian marriage: "This is a great sacrament; but I speak in Christ and in the Church."

Reflection: Sexuality within a sacramental marriage is the healthy context and a source of cure for those dealing with sexual trauma, abuse, rejection and pain. The Sacramental marital relationship is the primary place where children can be raised to become saints and find protection from evil and addictions. The sacramental marriage is a place where the suffering soul can experience healing, reconciliation, and unconditional love.

6.   Sacrament of Holy Orders Cure for the Addicted Soul.

   a.   Christ founded His Church as a supernatural society, the Kingdom of God. In this society there must be the power of ruling; and also the principles by which the members are to attain their supernatural end, viz.,supernatural truth, which is held by faith, and supernatural grace by which man is formally elevated to the supernatural order.

   b.   Thus, besides the power of jurisdiction, the Church has the power of teaching (*magisterium*) and the power of conferring grace (power of order). This power of order was committed by our Lord to His Apostles, who were to continue His work and to be His earthly representatives.

c. The first effect of the sacrament is an increase
   of sanctifying grace. With this, there is
   the sacramental grace which makes the recipient a fit
   and holy minister in the discharge of his office. As
   the duties of God's ministers are manifold and onerous, it
   is in perfect accord with the rulings of God's
   Providence to confer a special grace on His ministers.
d. The dispensation of sacraments requires grace, and the
   rightful discharge of sacred offices presupposes a special
   degree of spiritual excellence. The
   external sacramental sign or the power of the order can be
   received and may exist without this grace. Grace is
   required for the worthy, not the valid, exercise of the
   power, which is immediately and inseparably connected
   with the priestly character.
e. The principal effect of the sacrament is the character,
   a spiritual and indelible mark impressed upon the soul, by
   which the recipient is distinguished from others,
   designated as a minister of Christ, and deputed and
   empowered to perform certain offices of Divine
   worship (Summa
   III.63.2). http://www.newadvent.org/cathen/11279a.htm

Scripture: (John 20:21).: "as the Father hath sent me, I also send you"

Reflections: One of the existential challenges is finding their vocational calling. Many addicts experience vocational crisis and are in conflict with themselves. The calling can be to marriage, the religious life, the celibate life, or to Holy Orders. It is the life of service that God will bless and anoint. In many cases addiction takes hold when there are conflicts between who a person feels they are and what they actually do for a living. Understanding purpose is key to the recovery process. Becoming immersed in God's calling is a key to living a healthy and fulfilled life. Vocation is not a job

7. **Sacrament of Reconciliation (Confession) as Cure for the Addicted Soul.**

   a. Penance is a sacrament of the New Law instituted by Christ in which forgiveness of sins committed after baptism is granted through the priest's absolution to those who with true sorrow confess their sins and promise to satisfy for the same.

   b. It is called a "sacrament" not simply a function or ceremony, because it is an outward sign instituted by Christ to impart grace to the soul. As an outward sign it comprises the actions of the penitent in presenting himself to the priest and accusing himself of his sins, and the actions of the priest in pronouncing absolution and imposing satisfaction.

   c. This whole procedure is usually called, from one of its parts, "confession", and it is said to take place in the "tribunal of penance", because it is a judicial process in which the penitent is at once the accuser, the person accused, and the witness, while the priest pronounces judgment and sentence.

   d. The grace conferred is deliverance from the guilt of sin and, in the case of mortal sin, from its eternal punishment; hence also reconciliation with God, justification.

   e. Finally, the confession is made not in the secrecy of the penitent's heart nor to a layman as friend and advocate, nor to a representative of human authority, but to a duly ordained priest with requisite jurisdiction and with the" power of the keys", i.e., the power to forgive sins which Christ granted to His Church. http://www.newadvent.org/cathen/11618c.htm

   Scripture:

   "Amen I say to you, whatsoever you shall bind upon earth, shall be bound also in heaven; and whatsoever you shall loose upon earth, shall be loosed also in heaven" (Matthew 18:18)

"As the Father hath sent me, I also send you. When he had said this, he breathed on them; and he said to them: Receive ye the Holy Ghost. Whose sins you shall forgive, they are forgiven them; and whose sins you shall retain, they are retained' (John 20:21-23).

Reflections: Secular professional counselors (psychologist, psychiatrist, therapist, physicians, lawyers) have functioned as "secular priests" in our modern society. They have become the confessional for those suffering emotional disorders and distress. People have an innate need to tell their story to another person to find resolve, justice or relief. There is a catharsis in expressing ones burdens to some whom they trust. The Sacrament of Reconciliation provides that sacred service to the person in need. The sacrament is especially powerful and healing to the person struggling with the trauma of addictions. They are absolved of the damaging effects of the addiction on their mortal souls. They are giving the hope of reconciling with God and with others whom they have injured.

Practical Suggestions for Addiction Recovery using Roman Catholic Theology

1. Get a complete medical examination.

2. Recommit to your Baptismal promises.

3. Commit to Daily Prayer (examples):
   a. Morning offering
   b. Angelus
   c. Liturgy of the Hours
   d. Rosary
   e. Prayer of Humility
   f. Daily examination of conscience
   g. Novenas

4. Prepare for and receive the Sacrament of Reconciliation (at least monthly)

5. Attend Daily Mass as often as possible

6. Go to Adoration weekly

7. Find a Roman Catholic Spiritual advisor and meet monthly

8. Experience a Catholic Retreat (examples):
    a. Consider making a Cursillo or ACTS weekend
    b. Silent retreat
    c. Catholic Conferences (Mens, Womens, or Family Conferences)
    d. Participate in Parish Missions.

9. Wear a Benedictine Medal or Crucifix and get it blessed by a Priest. It is a protection from the presence and influences of evil

10. Consider a Marian Consecration: As Roman Catholics we believe those that have died in particular the saints are aware of living humans and the struggles we have, They actively prayer for us. We believe we can ask the saints in heaven to prayer for us. A devotion to the Blessed Mother of Christ Mary is a sample spiritual exercise. We can ask her to pray for us and for those we love.

11. Join and actively attend a weekly support group
    a. 12- Step Program
    b. Celebrate Recovery
    c. Faith based support group

12. Consider faith based individual, marital or family counseling.

13. Read or listen to faith based Roman Catholic resources weekly.
   .
14. Participate in New Evangelism and actively share your spiritual experience with others who may be struggling.

Statistics on Drug Usage:

According to SAMHSA (2007):

- Marijuana was the most commonly used illicit drug in 2006, accounting for 72.8 percent of illicit drug use.
- In 2006, there were 2.4 million cocaine users, a figure that remained the same from 2005 but was an increase from 2002 (at 2.0 million).
- The number of heroin users increased from 136,000 in 2005 to 338,000 in 2006, and the corresponding prevalence rate increased from 0.06 to 0.14 percent.
- The most widely used substance continues to be alcohol. In 2006, heavy drinking was reported by 6.9 percent of the population (17 million people), while binge drinking was reported by 23 percent (57 million people).

https://www.childwelfare.gov/pubs/factsheets/parentalsubabuse.cfm#1

The Oxford Group (12Step.com):

From "A First Century Christian Fellowship" to "Moral Re-Armament, The Oxford Group had many faces throughout the 20th Century. The Oxford Group began under the leadership of Frank Buchman, a Lutheran Minister and attained world wide fame by the time World War 2 began. From "A First Century Christian

Fellowship" to "Moral Re-Armament, The Oxford Group had many faces throughout the 20th Century. The Oxford Group began under the leadership of Frank Buchman, a Lutheran Minister and attained world wide fame by the time World War 2 began.

The Oxford Group had many different teachings, but the most important teachings as espoused by Frank Buchman can be summarized in 4 points:

1. Absolute Honesty

2. Absolute Purity

3. Absolute Unselfishness

4. Absolute Love

http://www.12step.com/oxfordgroup.html

Bill Wilson attended the Oxford Group in New York between 1932 and 1933 and many times directly connected the 12 Steps to his attendance at Oxford Group meetings. In fact, Rev. Sam Shoemaker, Buchman's partner personally assisted Bill Wilson's writing of Alcohol Anonymous' "The Big Book." Despite these clear connections, Bill Wilson drifted away from the Oxford Group's "Buchmanism" by mainstreaming the thoughts and ideologies of A.A. and the 12 Steps.

Bill Wilson didn't plan on becoming the creator of one of the most influential organizations to have been established in America in the 20th Century. In fact, when he had his first drink when he was a 22 year old, the last thing he was thinking was becoming an alcoholic and hitting bottom 17 years later, only to transform himself and countless others into sober individuals.

For 17 years after his first drink Bill Wilson suffered from alcoholism. By 1933 his once promising career as a Wall Street investor was no more and he and his wife found themselves in poverty. When through a friend he began to attend Frank

Buchman's Oxford Group, the meetings gave him the strength to sober up.

It wasn't until the end of the next five months of sobriety in a hotel lobby in Akron, Ohio that Wilson's "religious experience" and transformation occurred. Bill Wilson stood in that hotel lobby in Akron, Ohio after a blown business deal wanting a drink, but instead his religious epiphany led him to help others and from small groups Alcoholics Anonymous was born.

Bill Wilson achieved success through being the "anonymous celebrity." Early on in his transformation from lonely alcoholic to the humble leader, Wilson wrote and developed the 12 Traditions and 12 Steps, which ultimately developed as the core piece of thought behind Alcoholics Anonymous. After some time he developed the "Big Book," based on his teachings and understandings from his support groups and the 12 Steps. Bill Wilson not only preached support groups based on anonymity, he lived by attending his own groups as Bill W. Wilson remained Bill W. until 1971, the year he died.
 http://www.12step.com/directory/treatment-centers/treatment-centers

12- Step Statistics 2008: http://www.12step.com/statistics.html
- Of those in their first month of AA meetings, 26% will still be attending at he end of that year.
- Of those in their fourth month of AA meeting attendance (i.e. have stayed beyond 90-days) 56% will still be attending AA at the end of that year.
- The 2004 Survey showed an increase in the length of sobriety over the 2001 Survey (as has every triennial survey since 1983).
- As of the 2004 Survey, long-term AA sobriety was so prevalent that the "Greater Than Five Years" range of previous surveys was subdivided into: 5-10 Years (14%) , >10 Years (36%), > 5 Years (50%).

- For growth of AA sobriety ranges, the 1983 Survey showed 25% of AA members sober over 5 years and the 2004 Survey showed 50% of AA members sober over 5 years.
- For growth of AA sobriety averages, the 1983 Survey found the average AA member sober for 4 years and the 2004 Survey found the average AA member sober for more than 8 years.

Sacrament of Baptism Prayer:

Then the Celebrant asks the following questions of the candidates who
can speak for themselves, and of the parents and godparents who speak
on behalf of the infants and younger children

Question Do you renounce Satan and all the spiritual forces of wickedness that rebel against God?

Answer I renounce them.

Question Do you renounce the evil powers of this world which corrupt and destroy the creatures of God?

Answer I renounce them.

Question Do you renounce all sinful desires that draw you from the love of God?

Answer I renounce them.

Question Do you turn to Jesus Christ and accept him as your Savior?

Answer I do.

Question Do you put your whole trust in his grace and love?

Answer   I do.

http://www.bcponline.org/Baptism/holybaptism.html

Catholic Prayer: Blessing of the Medal of St. Benedict

V. *Our help is in the name of the Lord.* **R.** Who made heaven and earth.

In the name of God the Father + almighty, who made heaven and earth, the seas and all that is in them, I exorcise these medals against the power and attacks of the evil one. May all who use these medals devoutly be blessed with health of soul and body. In the name of the Father + almighty, of his Son + Jesus Christ our Lord, and of the Holy + Spirit the Paraclete, and in the love of the same Lord Jesus Christ who will come on the last day to judge the living and the dead, and the world by fire. Amen.

Let us pray. Almighty God, the boundless source of all good things, we humbly, ask that, through the intercession of St. Benedict, you pour out your blessings + upon these medals. May those who use them devoutly and earnestly strive to perform good works be blessed by you with health of soul and body, the grace of a holy life, and remission of the temporal punishment due to sin. May they also, with the help of your merciful love, resist the temptations of the evil one and strive to exercise true charity and justice toward all, so that one day they may appear sinless and holy in your sight. This we ask through Christ our Lord. **R.** Amen.

O Almighty God, the Giver of all good gifts, we humbly beseech Thee that Thou wouldst bestow, through the intercession of the holy

Father St. Benedict, Thy blessing upon these Medals, their letters and characters designed by Thee, that all who wear them and strive to perform good works may obtain health of body and soul, the grace of salvation, the indulgences conceded to us, and by the assistance of Thy mercy, escape the snares and deceptions of the devil and appear holy and stainless in Thy sight. Through Christ Our Lord. Amen

Begone, Satan!
Suggest not vain things to me.
Evil is the cup thou offerest;
Drink thou thine own poison.

http://www.olrl.org/sacramental/benedictmedal.shtml

Prayer to Mary, Undoer of Knots

Virgin Mary, Mother of fair love, Mother who never refuses to come to the aid of a child in need, Mother whose hands never cease to serve your beloved children because they are moved by the divine love and immense mercy that exists in your heart, cast your compassionate eyes upon me and see the snarl of knots that exist in my life. You know very well how desperate I am, my pain, and how I am bound by these knots. Mary, Mother to whom God entrusted the undoing of the knots in the lives of his children, I entrust into your hands the ribbon of my life. No one, not even the Evil One himself, can take it away from your precious care. In your hands there is no knot that cannot be undone. Powerful Mother, by your grace and intercessory power with Your Son and My Liberator, Jesus, take into your hands today this knot.

[Mention your request here]

I beg you to undo it for the glory of God, once for all. You are my hope. O my Lady, you are the only consolation God gives me, the fortification of my feeble strength, the enrichment of my destitution,

and, with Christ, the freedom from my chains. Hear my plea.
Keep me, guide me, protect me, o safe refuge!

Mary, Undoer of Knots, pray for me.

The Litany of Humility Prayer

O Jesus! meek and humble of heart, Hear me.
From the desire of being esteemed,
Deliver me, Jesus. (repeat after each line)
From the desire of being loved,
From the desire of being extolled,
From the desire of being honored,
From the desire of being praised,
From the desire of being preferred to others,
From the desire of being consulted,
From the desire of being approved,
From the fear of being humiliated,
From the fear of being despised,
From the fear of suffering rebukes,
From the fear of being calumniated,
From the fear of being forgotten,
From the fear of being ridiculed,
From the fear of being wronged,
From the fear of being suspected,
That others may be loved more than I,
Jesus, grant me the grace to desire it. (repeat after each line)
That others may be esteemed more than I ,
That, in the opinion of the world,
others may increase and I may decrease,
That others may be chosen and I set aside,
That others may be praised and I unnoticed,
That others may be preferred to me in everything,
That others may become holier than I, provided that I may become
as holy as I should,

Scriptures Dealing with Addictions:

1 Corinthians 10:13 ESV / 835 helpful votes

No temptation has overtaken you that is not common to man. God is faithful, and he will not let you be tempted beyond your ability, but with the temptation he will also provide the way of escape, that you may be able to endure it.

1 Peter 5:8 ESV / 380 helpful votes

Be sober-minded; be watchful. Your adversary the devil prowls around like a roaring lion, seeking someone to devour.

James 1:12-15 ESV / 312 helpful votes

Blessed is the man who remains steadfast under trial, for when he has stood the test he will receive the crown of life, which God has promised to those who love him. Let no one say when he is tempted, "I am being tempted by God," for God cannot be tempted with evil, and he himself tempts no one. But each person is tempted when he is lured and enticed by his own desire. Then desire when it has conceived gives birth to sin, and sin when it is fully grown brings forth death.

1 John 2:16 ESV / 225 helpful votes

For all that is in the world—the desires of the flesh and the desires of the eyes and pride in possessions—is not from the Father but is from the world.

1 Corinthians 15:33 ESV / 197 helpful votes

Do not be deceived: "Bad company ruins good morals."

James 4:7 ESV / 179 helpful votes

Submit yourselves therefore to God. Resist the devil, and he will flee from you.

Galatians 5:19-21 ESV / 167 helpful votes

Now the works of the flesh are evident: sexual immorality, impurity, sensuality, idolatry, sorcery, enmity, strife, jealousy, fits of anger, rivalries, dissensions, divisions, envy, drunkenness, orgies, and things like these. I warn you, as I warned you before, that those who do such things will not inherit the kingdom of God.

1 Corinthians 6:12 ESV / 164 helpful votes

"All things are lawful for me," but not all things are helpful. "All things are lawful for me," but I will not be enslaved by anything.

1 Peter 2:11 ESV / 140 helpful votes

Beloved, I urge you as sojourners and exiles to abstain from the passions of the flesh, which wage war against your soul.

1 Peter 5:10 ESV / 135 helpful votes

And after you have suffered a little while, the God of all grace, who has called you to his eternal glory in Christ, will himself restore, confirm, strengthen, and establish you.

Proverbs 20:1 ESV / 128 helpful votes

Wine is a mocker, strong drink a brawler, and whoever is led astray by it is not wise.

Romans 13:14 ESV / 116 helpful votes

But put on the Lord Jesus Christ, and make no provision for the flesh, to gratify its desires.

1 Corinthians 6:18 ESV / 108 helpful votes

Flee from sexual immorality. Every other sin a person commits is outside the body, but the sexually immoral person sins against his own body.

Psalm 50:15 ESV / 105 helpful votes

And call upon me in the day of trouble; I will deliver you, and you shall glorify me."

Proverbs 6:27 ESV / 94 helpful votes

Can a man carry fire next to his chest and his clothes not be burned?

Matthew 6:13 ESV / 90 helpful votes

And lead us not into temptation, but deliver us from evil.

Romans 5:3-5 ESV / 83 helpful votes

More than that, we rejoice in our sufferings, knowing that suffering produces endurance, and endurance produces character, and character produces hope, and hope does not put us to shame, because God's love has been poured into our hearts through the Holy Spirit who has been given to us.

John 8:36 ESV / 81 helpful votes

So if the Son sets you free, you will be free indeed.

1 John 3:8 ESV / 75 helpful votes

Whoever makes a practice of sinning is of the devil, for the devil has been sinning from the beginning. The reason the Son of God appeared was to destroy the works of the devil.

1 Corinthians 6:9-11 ESV / 71 helpful votes

Or do you not know that the unrighteous will not inherit the kingdom of God? Do not be deceived: neither the sexually immoral, nor idolaters, nor adulterers, nor men who practice homosexuality, nor thieves, nor the greedy, nor drunkards, nor revilers, nor swindlers will inherit the kingdom of God. And such were some of you. But you were washed, you were sanctified, you were justified in the name of the Lord Jesus Christ and by the Spirit of our God.

Galatians 5:16 ESV / 69 helpful votes

But I say, walk by the Spirit, and you will not gratify the desires of the flesh.

Philippians 4:4-7 ESV / 67 helpful votes

Rejoice in the Lord always; again I will say, Rejoice. Let your reasonableness be known to everyone. The Lord is at hand; do not be anxious about anything, but in everything by prayer and supplication with thanksgiving let your requests be made known to God. And the peace of God, which surpasses all understanding, will guard your hearts and your minds in Christ Jesus.

Titus 2:12 ESV / 63 helpful votes

Training us to renounce ungodliness and worldly passions, and to live self-controlled, upright, and godly lives in the present age,

2 Peter 2:19 ESV / 59 helpful votes

They promise them freedom, but they themselves are slaves of corruption. For whatever overcomes a person, to that he is enslaved.

Romans 8:5-6 ESV / 52 helpful votes

For those who live according to the flesh set their minds on the things of the flesh, but those who live according to the Spirit set their minds on the things of the Spirit. For to set the mind on the flesh is death, but to set the mind on the Spirit is life and peace.

Romans 8:1-2 ESV / 49 helpful votes

There is therefore now no condemnation for those who are in Christ Jesus. For the law of the Spirit of life has set you free in Christ Jesus from the law of sin and death.

1 Corinthians 6:11 ESV / 41 helpful votes

And such were some of you. But you were washed, you were sanctified, you were justified in the name of the Lord Jesus Christ and by the Spirit of our God.

Colossians 3:5 ESV / 40 helpful votes

Put to death therefore what is earthly in you: sexual immorality, impurity, passion, evil desire, and covetousness, which is idolatry.

Galatians 5:24-25 ESV / 39 helpful votes

And those who belong to Christ Jesus have crucified the flesh with its passions and desires. If we live by the Spirit, let us also walk by the Spirit.

Ephesians 5:18 ESV / 35 helpful votes

And do not get drunk with wine, for that is debauchery, but be filled with the Spirit,

Proverbs 23:20 ESV / 35 helpful votes

Be not among drunkards or among gluttonous eaters of meat,

Psalm 121:1-2 ESV / 33 helpful votes

A Song of Ascents. I lift up my eyes to the hills. From where does my help come? My help comes from theLord, who made heaven and earth.

James 1:2-3 ESV / 32 helpful votes

Count it all joy, my brothers, when you meet trials of various kinds, for you know that the testing of your faith produces steadfastness.

Hebrews 4:15-16 ESV / 32 helpful votes

For we do not have a high priest who is unable to sympathize with our weaknesses, but one who in every respect has been tempted as we are, yet without sin. Let us then with confidence draw near to the throne of grace, that we may receive mercy and find grace to help in time of need.

Matthew 5:28 ESV / 29 helpful votes

But I say to you that everyone who looks at a woman with lustful intent has already committed adultery with her in his heart.

2 Corinthians 4:16-18 ESV / 28 helpful votes

So we do not lose heart. Though our outer self is wasting away, our inner self is being renewed day by day. For this light momentary affliction is preparing for us an eternal weight of glory beyond all comparison, as we look not to the things that are seen but to the things that are unseen. For the things that are seen are transient, but the things that are unseen are eternal.

1 Corinthians 5:11 ESV / 27 helpful votes

But now I am writing to you not to associate with anyone who bears the name of brother if he is guilty of sexual immorality or greed, or is an idolater, reviler, drunkard, or swindler—not even to eat with such a one.

John 3:16-17 ESV / 27 helpful votes

"For God so loved the world, that he gave his only Son, that whoever believes in him should not perish but have eternal life. For

God did not send his Son into the world to condemn the world, but in order that the world might be saved through him.

Matthew 18:7 ESV / 27 helpful votes

"Woe to the world for temptations to sin! For it is necessary that temptations come, but woe to the one by whom the temptation comes!

Isaiah 40:31 ESV / 27 helpful votes

But they who wait for the Lord shall renew their strength; they shall mount up with wings like eagles; they shall run and not be weary; they shall walk and not faint.

1 Corinthians 3:17 ESV / 26 helpful votes

If anyone destroys God's temple, God will destroy him. For God's temple is holy, and you are that temple.

Philippians 4:13 ESV / 25 helpful votes

I can do all things through him who strengthens me.

Galatians 5:1 ESV / 24 helpful votes

For freedom Christ has set us free; stand firm therefore, and do not submit again to a yoke of slavery.

Romans 13:13-14 ESV / 23 helpful votes

Let us walk properly as in the daytime, not in orgies and drunkenness, not in sexual immorality and sensuality, not in quarreling and jealousy. But put on the Lord Jesus Christ, and make no provision for the flesh, to gratify its desires.

Romans 6:6-7 ESV / 23 helpful votes

We know that our old self was crucified with him in order that the body of sin might be brought to nothing, so that we would no longer be enslaved to sin. For one who has died has been set free from sin.

Ephesians 5:5 ESV / 21 helpful votes

For you may be sure of this, that everyone who is sexually immoral or impure, or who is covetous (that is, an idolater), has no inheritance in the kingdom of Christ and God.

Romans 6:17-18 ESV / 21 helpful votes

But thanks be to God, that you who were once slaves of sin have become obedient from the heart to the standard of teaching to which you were committed, and, having been set free from sin, have become slaves of righteousness.

Matthew 5:29-30 ESV / 21 helpful votes

If your right eye causes you to sin, tear it out and throw it away. For it is better that you lose one of your members than that your whole body be thrown into hell. And if your right hand causes you to sin, cut it off and throw it away. For it is better that you lose one of your members than that your whole body go into hell.

Jude 1:24-25 ESV / 20 helpful votes

Now to him who is able to keep you from stumbling and to present you blameless before the presence of his glory with great joy, to the only God, our Savior, through Jesus Christ our Lord, be glory, majesty, dominion, and authority, before all time and now and forever. Amen.

Luke 6:20-49 ESV / 20 helpful votes

And he lifted up his eyes on his disciples, and said: "Blessed are you who are poor, for yours is the kingdom of God. "Blessed are you who are hungry now, for you shall be satisfied. "Blessed are you who weep now, for you shall laugh. "Blessed are you when people hate you and when they exclude you and revile you and spurn your name as evil, on account of the Son of Man! Rejoice in that day, and leap for joy, for behold, your reward is great in heaven; for so their fathers did to the prophets. "But woe to you who are rich, for you have received your consolation.

Isaiah 5:11 ESV / 20 helpful votes

Woe to those who rise early in the morning, that they may run after strong drink, who tarry late into the evening as wine inflames them!

Luke 7:47 ESV / 19 helpful votes

Therefore I tell you, her sins, which are many, are forgiven—for she loved much. But he who is forgiven little, loves little."

Romans 14:21 ESV / 18 helpful votes

It is good not to eat meat or drink wine or do anything that causes your brother to stumble.

Romans 8:12-13 ESV / 18 helpful votes

So then, brothers, we are debtors, not to the flesh, to live according to the flesh. For if you live according to the flesh you will die, but if by the Spirit you put to death the deeds of the body, you will live.

Romans 6:16 ESV / 18 helpful votes

Do you not know that if you present yourselves to anyone as obedient slaves, you are slaves of the one whom you obey, either of sin, which leads to death, or of obedience, which leads to righteousness?

1 Peter 4:10 ESV / 17 helpful votes

As each has received a gift, use it to serve one another, as good stewards of God's varied grace:

Hebrews 13:4 ESV / 17 helpful votes

Let marriage be held in honor among all, and let the marriage bed be undefiled, for God will judge the sexually immoral and adulterous.

1 Corinthians 3:16 ESV / 17 helpful votes

Do you not know that you are God's temple and that God's Spirit dwells in you?

Jeremiah 29:11 ESV / 17 helpful votes

For I know the plans I have for you, declares the Lord, plans for welfare and not for evil, to give you a future and a hope.

Ephesians 5:18-20 ESV / 16 helpful votes

And do not get drunk with wine, for that is debauchery, but be filled with the Spirit, addressing one another in psalms and hymns and spiritual songs, singing and making melody to the Lord with your heart, giving thanks always and for everything to God the Father in the name of our Lord Jesus Christ,

Romans 6:6 ESV / 16 helpful votes

We know that our old self was crucified with him in order that the body of sin might be brought to nothing, so that we would no longer be enslaved to sin.

Matthew 4:1-11 ESV / 16 helpful votes

Then Jesus was led up by the Spirit into the wilderness to be tempted by the devil. And after fasting forty days and forty nights, he was hungry. And the tempter came and said to him, "If you are the Son of God, command these stones to become loaves of bread." But he answered, "It is written, "'Man shall not live by bread alone, but by every word that comes from the mouth of God.'" Then the devil took him to the holy city and set him on the pinnacle of the temple

1 Corinthians 8:9 ESV / 14 helpful votes

But take care that this right of yours does not somehow become a stumbling block to the weak.

Matthew 26:29 ESV / 14 helpful votes

I tell you I will not drink again of this fruit of the vine until that day when I drink it new with you in my Father's kingdom."

Matthew 5:13-16 ESV / 14 helpful votes

"You are the salt of the earth, but if salt has lost its taste, how shall its saltiness be restored? It is no longer good for anything except to be thrown out and trampled under people's feet. "You are the light of the world. A city set on a hill cannot be hidden. Nor do people light a lamp and put it under a basket, but on a stand, and it gives light to all in the house. In the same way, let your light shine before others, so that they may see your good works and give glory to your Father who is in heaven.

Romans 12:2 ESV / 13 helpful votes

Do not be conformed to this world, but be transformed by the renewal of your mind, that by testing you may discern what is the will of God, what is good and acceptable and perfect.

Romans 7:14-25 ESV / 13 helpful votes

For we know that the law is spiritual, but I am of the flesh, sold under sin. For I do not understand my own actions. For I do not do what I want, but I do the very thing I hate. Now if I do what I do not want, I agree with the law, that it is good. So now it is no longer I who do it, but sin that dwells within me. For I know that nothing good dwells in me, that is, in my flesh. For I have the desire to do what is right, but not the ability to carry it out.

Hosea 4:11 ESV / 13 helpful votes

Whoredom, wine, and new wine, which take away the understanding.

Romans 14:20-21 ESV / 12 helpful votes

Do not, for the sake of food, destroy the work of God. Everything is indeed clean, but it is wrong for anyone to make another stumble by what he eats. It is good not to eat meat or drink wine or do anything that causes your brother to stumble.

Proverbs 1:1-33 ESV / 12 helpful votes

The proverbs of Solomon, son of David, king of Israel: To know wisdom and instruction, to understand words of insight, to receive instruction in wise dealing, in righteousness, justice, and equity; to give prudence to the simple, knowledge and discretion to the youth— Let the wise hear and increase in learning, and the one who understands obtain guidance,

Philippians 3:12-14 ESV / 11 helpful votes

Not that I have already obtained this or am already perfect, but I press on to make it my own, because Christ Jesus has made me his own. Brothers, I do not consider that I have made it my own. But one thing I do: forgetting what lies behind and straining forward to what lies ahead, I press on toward the goal for the prize of the upward call of God in Christ Jesus.

Jeremiah 17:5-11 ESV / 10 helpful votes

Thus says the Lord: "Cursed is the man who trusts in man and makes flesh his strength, whose heart turns away from the Lord. He is like a shrub in the desert, and shall not see any good come. He shall dwell in the parched places of the wilderness, in an uninhabited salt land. "Blessed is the man who trusts in the Lord, whose trust is the Lord. He is like a tree planted by water, that sends out its roots by the stream, and does not fear when heat comes, for its leaves remain green, and is not anxious in the year of drought, for it does not cease to bear fruit." The heart is deceitful above all things, and desperately sick; who can understand it?

Proverbs 23:29-35 ESV / 10 helpful votes

Who has woe? Who has sorrow? Who has strife? Who has complaining? Who has wounds without cause? Who has redness of eyes? Those who tarry long over wine; those who go to try mixed wine. Do not look at wine when it is red, when it sparkles in the cup and goes down smoothly. In the end it bites like a serpent and stings like an adder. Your eyes will see strange things, and your heart utter perverse things.

Psalm 104:14-15 ESV / 9 helpful votes

You cause the grass to grow for the livestock and plants for man to cultivate, that he may bring forth food from the earth and wine to gladden the heart of man, oil to make his face shine and bread to strengthen man's heart.

2 Timothy 2:26 ESV / 4 helpful votes

And they may come to their senses and escape from the snare of the devil, after being captured by him to do his will.

2 Timothy 2:22 ESV / 4 helpful votes

So flee youthful passions and pursue righteousness, faith, love, and peace, along with those who call on the Lord from a pure heart.

2 Corinthians 11:14 ESV / 4 helpful votes

And no wonder, for even Satan disguises himself as an angel of light.

Luke 22:41-46 ESV / 4 helpful votes

And he withdrew from them about a stone's throw, and knelt down and prayed, saying, "Father, if you are willing, remove this cup from me. Nevertheless, not my will, but yours, be done." And there appeared to him an angel from heaven, strengthening him. And being in an agony he prayed more earnestly; and his sweat became like great drops of blood falling down to the ground. And when he rose from prayer, he came to the disciples and found them sleeping for sorrow,

Psalm 19:13 ESV / 4 helpful votes

Keep back your servant also from presumptuous sins; let them not have dominion over me! Then I shall be blameless, and innocent of great transgression.

Proverbs 23:2 ESV / 3 helpful votes

And put a knife to your throat if you are given to appetite.

St. Maximilian Kolbe is the patron Saint of Addicts

#1 A Novena to Saint Maximilian Kolbe for the Grace to be Freed from Addiction (pray this 9 days in a row)

Saint Maximilian Kolbe, your life of love and labor for souls was sacrificed amid the horrors of a concentration camp and hastened to its end by an injection of a deadly drug.

Look with compassion upon (NAME OF PERSON) who is now entrapped in addiction to drugs/alcohol and whom I now recommend to your powerful intercession. Having offered your own life to preserve that of a family man, I turn to you with trust, confident that you will understand and help.

Obtain for me the grace never to withhold my love and understanding, or to fail in persevering prayer that the enslaving bonds of addiction may be broken and that full health may be restored to him, whom I love.

I will never cease to be grateful to God who has helped me and heard your prayer for me.

Amen.

http://www.marytown.com/content/novena-to-st-maximilian-kolbe

Sources

Biblical References to Addictions

http://www.openbible.info/topics/addiction

http://godsbreath.net/2011/12/02/addiction-bible-verses/

http://www.bradhambrick.com/bibleversesonaddiction/

http://www.bibletools.org/index.cfm/fuseaction/Topical.show/RTD/cgg/ID/884/Addiction-Sin.htm

Addiction Definition:

http://www.asam.org/for-the-public/definition-of-addiction

http://www.aamft.org/imis15/content/consumer_updates/sexual_addiction.aspx

Statistics on Addictions:

http://www.helpguide.org/harvard/addiction_hijacks_brain.htm

http://www.drugabuse.gov/related-topics/trends-statistics.

Sex Addiction:

http://www.aamft.org/imis15/content/consumer_updates/sexual_addiction.aspx

Compulsive Eating Disorders:

http://www.anad.org/get-information/about-eating-disorders/eating-disorders-statistics/

The Drug Trafficking:

https://www.unodc.org/unodc/en/drug-trafficking/index.html

http://drugabuse.com/library/workplace-drug-abuse/

The Sex Trafficking in the United States:

http://thecoveringhouse.org/act/resources-2/sex-trafficking-statistics-source-documentation/
http://www.dui.com/
http://www.divorcelawfirms.com/resources/divorce/divorce-children/the-link-between-addiction-divorce

Drug Related Prison Offenses:

http://www.huffingtonpost.com/2013/04/08/drug-war-mass-incarceration_n_3034310.html

http://www.samhsa.gov/data/2k13/NSDUH036/SR036SubstanceUse
Dropouts.htm

Child Abuse:

https://www.childwelfare.gov/pubs/factsheets/parentalsubabuse.cfm
#1

Work force Impact:

http://drugabuse.com/library/workplace-drug-abuse/

Addiction and the Brain:

http://www.helpguide.org/harvard/addiction_hijacks_brain.htm

Psychological Impact:

. http://www.helpguide.org/harvard/addiction_hijacks_brain.htm

Sociological Impact:

http://www.helpguide.org/harvard/addiction_hijacks_brain.htm

Definitions of Spirituality:

http://www.psychologytoday.com/basics/spirituality
http://dictionary.reference.com/browse/spirituality
https://archive.org/stream/SpiritualTheologyByFr.JordanAumannO.p
/AumannO.p.SpiritualTheologyall_djvu.txt

The 12- Step Philosophy and Program (12Step.com):

http://www.12step.com/history.html

What are the 12 Steps and their Scriptural references?

http://12step.org/bible/step-12-scriptures.html

What is the Definition of Grace?

. http://www.newadvent.org/cathen/06701a.htm

Definition of Sacraments (New Advent.org):

http://www.newadvent.org/cathen/13295a.htm.

Sacrament of Baptism as Cure for the Addicted soul.

http://www.newadvent.org/cathen/02258b.htm

Sacrament of Confirmation as Cure:

http://www.newadvent.org/cathen/04215b.htm

Sacrament of the Eucharist as Cure:

http://www.newadvent.org/cathen/05584a.htm

Sacrament of the Extreme Unction (Anointing of the Sick) as Cure

. http://www.newadvent.org/cathen/05716a.htm

Sacrament of Marriage as Cure :

http://www.newadvent.org/cathen/09707a.htm

Sacrament of Holy Orders as Cure

http://www.newadvent.org/cathen/11279a.htm

Sacrament of Reconciliation (Confession) as Cure:

http://www.newadvent.org/cathen/11618c.htm

Understanding Addiction and Evil: Finding Healing Through the 12 Steps and Spirituality

Quiz

By

Kevin Stephenson. M.Div. M.A. LPC-S. BCC.

(A Grade of 60% or greater needed to obtain Oklahoma LPC/LMFT CEU Certificate)

1. The following were consider ancient Greek philosophers:
   a. Socrates, Plato and Aristotle
   b. Plato, Aristotle and St. Augustine
   c. Socrates, Saint Augustine, St Thomas Aquinas
   d. Plato, St. Augustine, St. Thomas Aquinas
2. _____ is experienced when people freely choose to act against the moral order.
   a. Physical Evil
   b. Moral Evil
   c. Metaphysical Evil
3. Addiction does not have a strong emotional and physical component that creates a high level of distress if not fulfilled.
   a. True
   b. False

4. Abuse of tobacco, alcohol, and illicit drugs is costly to the United Sates, exacting over $600 billion annually in costs related to crime
   a. True
   b. False.
5. This addiction costs Healthcare: $30 Billion and overall: $235 Billion
   a. Tobacco
   b. Alcohol
   c. Narcotics
6. Only 20% of the world's illegal drugs are consumed by American drug users.
   a. True
   b. False
7. 2.2 million Americans are in prison or jail for drug related offenses.
   More than half of federal prisoners are incarcerated for drug crimes in 2010.
   a. True
   b. False
8. A 2007 study done by the Rand Corporation found that alcohol was the single most significant factor in early divorce among young couples.
   a. True
   b. False

9. Substance use rates among 12th grade aged youths who had dropped out of school were lower than among those who were still in school; for example, 22.4 percent of dropouts were current cigarette users compared with 56.8 percent of those still in school.
   a. True
   b. False
10. Fetal alcohol spectrum disorders (FASD) are among the most well-known consequences, affecting an estimated 40,000

infants born each year. Oklahoma had almost 11,000 kids in state custody—mostly because of illicit drug issues
    a. True
    b. False

11. 10 to 20 percent of American workers who die at work have a positive result when tested for drugs or alcohol. A study by OSHA states that the most dangerous occupations, such as mining and construction, also have the highest rates of drug use by their employees.
    a. True
    b. False

12. The continued use of ETOH or poly substance excessively in a way that damages one or more area of a person's life. The areas affected are mental, physical health, family life, social relationships, job and economic viability, creativity and spiritual wholeness is:
    a. Alcoholism:
    b. A progressive compulsive-addictive illness
    c. Compulsive

13. Psychologically the desire to abuse ETOH or Poly Substance is driven at an unconscious level. To the degree a person reports being out of control with the substance abuse.
    a. Alcoholism:
    b. A progressive compulsive-addictive illness
    c. Compulsive

14. It is a physiological adaptation of a person to the ETOH/Poly Sub that creates acute distress and intense cravings when the abuse stops.
    a. Addictive
    b. Progressive
    c. Problem Drinking

15. When an illness progresses in predicable stages and if not treated will result in irreversible dysfunction and eventually death. Increased dependence or loss of control can progress over a period of 5 to 15 years.

a. Problem Drinking
b. Progressive
c. Chronic Alcoholism

16. Is an all-inclusive term which can include non- addictive ETOH behavior. An example would be driving an automotive while under the influence of ETOH. Or engaging in self destructive behavior (unprotected sexual behavior or altercations with strangers) while under the influence of ETOH.
    a. Problem Drinking:
    b. Chronic Alcoholism
    c. Steady Drinker with Binges
17. An advanced stage in the illness where severe medical or psychiatric complications occur.
    a. Chronic Alcoholism
    b. Steady Drinker with Binges
    c. Periodic Alcoholic
18. Is the degree of personal or social disintegration a person has to experience before they seek outside help for the addiction:
    a. Plateau Alcoholic
    b. High or Low Bottom Alcoholics
    c. Recreational Drunkenness
19. Usually includes psychological problems that are present prior to the person abusing and becoming dependent on ETOH. ETOH is often utilized for its psychological pain numbing effects.
    a. Low Bottom Alcoholic
    b. Soil of Addiction

c. Pre-Alcoholics

20. Learned social and cultural behaviors may be a contributing factor. For example in Ireland and France there is a higher rate of ETOH abuse compared to other countries.
   a. Sociocultural
   b. Spiritual
   c. Both
   d. None of the above

21. Religious anxiety, fear of death, meaninglessness, unresolved guilt may contribute to ETOH abuse. Spiritual ETOH can falsely serve as a spiritual transcendences. ETOH addiction may serve as a form of idolatry.
   a. Sociocultural
   b. Spiritual
   c. Both
   d. None of the above

22. Sexual addiction is a serious problem in which one engages in persistent and escalating patterns of sexual behavior despite increasing negative consequences to one's self or others.
   a. True
   b. False

23. Approximately 300,000 children are at risk of being prostituted in the United States.
   a. True
   b. False

24. Up to 24 million people of all ages and genders suffer from an eating disorder (anorexia, bulimia and binge eating disorder) in the U.S.
   a. True
   b. False

25. Type 2 diabetes usually develops gradually over a number of years, beginning when muscle and other cells stop responding to insulin. This condition, known as insulin resistance, causes blood sugar and insulin levels to stay too low long after eating.

a. True

b. False

26. Diabetes remains the 7th leading cause of death in the United States in 2010, with 69,071 death certificates listing it as the underlying cause of death, and a total of 234,051 death certificates listing diabetes as an underlying or contributing cause of death.

    a. True

    b. False

27. 15.9% of this ethic group are diagnosed with diabetes

    a. Asian Americans

    b. Hispanics

    c. Non-Hispanic Black

    d. American Indians/Alaskan Natives

28. 13.2% of this ethic group are diagnosed with diabetes.

    a. Asian Americans

    b. Hispanics

    c. Non-Hispanic Black

    d. American Indians/Alaskan Natives

29. Annual Cost of Diabetes is:

    a. $245 billion:

    b. $176 billion

    c. $69 billion

30. In the brain, pleasure has a distinct signature: the release of the neurotransmitter _____ in the **nucleus accumbens**, a cluster of nerve cells lying underneath the cerebral cortex.

    a. Gluconate

    b. Norepinephrine

    c. Dopamine

    d. Serotonin

31. According to the current theory about addiction, **dopamine** interacts with another neurotransmitter _____ to take over the brain's system of reward-related learning.
    a. Gluconate
    b. Norepinephrine
    c. Dopamine
    d. Serotonin
32. Repeated exposure to an addictive substance or behavior causes nerve cells in the **nucleus accumbens** and the_____ (the area of the brain involved in planning and executing tasks) to communicate in a way that couples liking something with wanting it, in turn driving us to go after it.
    a. Brain Stem
    b. Prefrontal Cortex
    c. Hippocampus
    d. Cerebral Cortex
33. Addictive drugs, for example, can release _____ the amount of **dopamine** that natural rewards do, and they do it more quickly and more reliably. In a person who becomes addicted, brain receptors become overwhelmed.
    a. 1 to 3 times
    b. 4 to 6 times
    c. 2 to 10 times
    d. 7 to 11 times.
34. The human brain utilizes glucose (fuel/energy) and water (oxygen) to function. Glucose comes from carbohydrate foods. Carbohydrates are made up of complex sugars (vegetables, grains, cereals) and simple sugars (fruits, juice, milk). A depletion or abuse in any of these resources will result in:
    e. Poor cognition
    f. Inattention
    g. Memory problems/loss
    h. Cell damage or cell death.
    i. All the Above

j. None of the Above
35. Amino acids are the building block for many neurotransmitters.
    a. True
    b. False
36. Three amino acids that work with neurotransmitters are:
    a. Trypophan
    b. Taurine
    c. Tyrosine
    d. All the above
    e. None of the above

37. Neurotransmitters (help transport information through nerves) and proteins. They consist of:
    a. Dopamine, Serotonin,
    b. Norepinephrine, Epinephrine,
    c. Histamine. Dopamine
    d. All the above
    e. None of the above
38. _____gives the body a natural "high" when something good happens (sexual activity, exercise, achievements, etc). It is depleted by processed sugar, caffeine, alcohol, sleep deprivation, and some anti-depressants).
    a. Dopamine
    b. Serotonin
    c. Norepinephrine
    d. Epinephrine
39. _____ helps maintain mood levels, regulate the gastral intestinal track. It is depleted by alcohol, caffeine, nicotine, poor sunlight, exposure to heavy metals and pesticides. If elevated it can result in manic, psychotic behavior.
    a. Dopamine

b. Serotonin

c. Norepinephrine

d. Epinephrine

40. _____it helps suppress neuro inflammation, regulated glucose release, and regulated the endocrine system. It is responsible for fight/flight response, attention response, decision making and goal directed behavior.

    a. Dopamine

    b. Serotonin

    c. Norepinephrine

    d. Epinephrine

41. _____its depletions can result in low blood pressure, excessive salt through kidneys, weight loss and chronic fatigue. What helps is sea salt and exercise.

    a. Dopamine

    b. Serotonin

    c. Norepinephrine

    d. Epinephrine

42. _____it maintains vigilance and alertness. Elevated levels found in people suffering from schizophrenia. It is naturally found in meats and hard cheeses.

    a. Serotonin

    b. Norepinephrine

    c. Epinephrine

    d. Histamine.

43. Refined Sugars reduce food nutrients and aggravates food intolerances.

    a. True

    b. False

44. Food Dyes contribute to AHDA behaviors and allergies in children.

    a. True

    b. False

45. The _____ and the _____ store
information about environmental cues associated with the
desired substance, so that it can be located again.
   a. Hippocampus, Amygdala
   b. Amygdala, Cerebral Cortex
   c. Prefrontal Lobe, Cerebral Cortex
   d. None of the Above
46. Whenever the person encounters_____. A person
addicted to heroin may be in danger of relapse when he sees
a hypodermic needle.
   a. Thoughts
   b. Feelings
   c. Environmental cues
   d. None of the above
47. Utilization of medical detoxification regime (in patient
medical facility) that may be a few days until the patient is
stabilized. Assign a psychiatrics or internal medicine
physician to administer medication management with nursing
care. Then given a social worker or case manager to plan
after care treatment is called:
   a. Medical Intervention
   b. Psychological/ Behavioral Health Intervention
   c. Social workers and Case Managers
   d. Community of Faith
48. They are assigned a mental health counselor or psychologist
for one on one treatment. Work on the behavioral and
emotional factors that contribute to the compulsive addictive
behavior. These sessions can be three to eight meetings. It
also depends the philosophical orientation of the therapist.
Some relationships may continue for a few years describes:
   a. Medical Intervention
   b. Psychological/ Behavioral Health Intervention
   c. Social workers and Case Managers
   d. Group Therapy
49. Due to the severity of the addictive process on their
interpersonal relationships. They will need considerable
assistance in basic living sustenance. May become indigent
and homeless or have dependent children who need care and
assistance. Many are unemployed, disabled or considered un

employable due to criminal backgrounds. They are in need of considerable social assistance describes:
- a. Medical Intervention
- b. Psychological/ Behavioral Health Intervention
- c. Social workers and Case Managers
- d. Community of Faith

50. Support groups ran by professional clinicians with the same goals as individual counseling but with a greater focus on psychological educational materials are called:
- a. Medical Intervention
- b. Psychological/ Behavioral Health Intervention
- c. Social workers and Case Managers
- d. Group Therapy

51. A community organized around a common belief, creed, philosophical mindset or covenant. They provide counseling or pastoral care services to members of their particular community is called:
- a. Psychological/ Behavioral Health Intervention
- b. Community of Faith
- c. Group Therapy
- d. Self-Help Groups

52. These groups are directed by nonprofessionals and peers. Typically, the leaders are folks who have recovered or in the process of recovering from addictive disorders.
- a. Psychological/ Behavioral Health Intervention
- b. Community of Faith
- c. Group Therapy
- d. Self-Help Groups

53. Which definition is part of the Oxford Group's Five C's:
- a. Confidence
- b. Confession
- c. Conversion
- d. Continuance
- e. All the above

54. The Big Book of Alcoholics Anonymous in 1938 was founded by:
- a. Colonel Sanders
- b. Eleonore Roosevelt

    c. Bill Wilson

    d. W.C. Fields

55. The 12-Step Program itself is over_____ old,

    a. 20

    b. 50

    c. 70

    d. 100

56. We admit we are powerless over (addiction)—that our lives have become unmanageable is Step:

    a. 1

    b. 2

    c. 3

    d. 4

57. We make a decision to turn our will and our lives over to the care of God as we understand Him is Step:

    a. 1

    b. 2

    c. 3

    d. 4

58. We come to believe that a Power greater than ourselves can restore us to sanity is Step:

    a. 1

    b. 2

    c. 3

    d. 4

59. We admit to God, to ourselves, and to another human being the exact nature of our wrongs is Step:

    a. 5

    b. 6

    c. 7

    d. 8

60. We humbly ask Him to remove our shortcomings is Step:

    a. 5

    b. 6

    c. 7

      d. 8

61. We make a searching and fearless moral inventory of ourselves is Step:
      a. 2
      b. 3
      c. 4
      d. 5

62. We make direct amends to such people wherever possible, except when to do so would injure them or others is Step:
      a. 9
      b. 10
      c. 11
      d. 12

63. We seek through prayer and <u>meditation</u> to improve our conscious contact with God as we understand Him, praying only for knowledge of His Will for us and the power to carry that out is Step:
      a. 9
      b. 10
      c. 11
      d. 12

64. We are entirely ready to have God remove all these defects of character is Step:
      a. 5
      b. 6
      c. 7
      d. 8

65. Having had a spiritual awakening as the result of these steps, we try to carry this message to alcoholics, and to practice these principles in all our affairs.
      a. 9
      b. 10
      c. 11
      d. 12

66. We continue to take personal inventory and when we are wrong promptly admitted it is step:
      e. 9
      f. 10
      g. 11

h. 12
67. We make a list of all persons we have harmed, and become willing to make amends to them all.
   a. 5
   b. 6
   c. 7
   d. 8

Understanding Addiction and Evil: Finding Healing Through the 12 Steps and Spirituality

Quiz ANSWER KEY

1. The following were consider ancient Greek philosophers:
   a. Socrates, Plato and Aristotle
   b. Plato, Aristotle and St. Augustine
   c. Socrates, Saint Augustine, St Thomas Aquinas
   d. Plato, St. Augustine, St. Thomas Aquinas
2. _____ is experienced when people freely choose to act against the moral order.
   a. Physical Evil
   b. Moral Evil
   c. Metaphysical Evil
3. Addiction does not have a strong emotional and physical component that creates a high level of distress if not fulfilled.
   a. True
   b. False
4. Abuse of tobacco, alcohol, and illicit drugs is costly to the United Sates, exacting over $600 billion annually in costs related to crime
   a. True
   b. False.
5. This addiction costs Healthcare: $30 Billion and overall: $235 Billion
   a. Tobacco
   b. Alcohol
   c. Narcotics

6. Only 20% of the world's illegal drugs are consumed by American drug users.
   a. True
   b. False
7. 2.2 million Americans are in prison or jail for drug related offenses.
   More than half of federal prisoners are incarcerated for drug crimes in 2010.
   a. True
   b. False
8. A 2007 study done by the Rand Corporation found that alcohol was the single most significant factor in early divorce among young couples.
   a. True
   b. False
9. Substance use rates among 12th grade aged youths who had dropped out of school were lower than among those who were still in school; for example, 22.4 percent of dropouts were current cigarette users compared with 56.8 percent of those still in school.
   a. True
   b. False
10. Fetal alcohol spectrum disorders (FASD) are among the most well-known consequences, affecting an estimated 40,000 infants born each year. Oklahoma had almost 11,000 kids in state custody—mostly because of illicit drug issues
    a. True
    b. False
11. 10 to 20 percent of American workers who die at work have a positive result when tested for drugs or alcohol. A study by OSHA states that the most dangerous occupations, such as mining and construction, also have the highest rates of drug use by their employees.
    a. True
    b. False

12. The continued use of ETOH or poly substance excessively in a way that damages one or more area of a person's life. The areas affected are mental, physical health, family life, social relationships, job and economic viability, creativity and spiritual wholeness is:
    a. Alcoholism:
    b. **A progressive compulsive-addictive illness**
    c. Compulsive
13. Psychologically the desire to abuse ETOH or Poly Substance is driven at an unconscious level. To the degree a person reports being out of control with the substance abuse.
    a. Alcoholism:
    b. A progressive compulsive-addictive illness
    c. **Compulsive**
14. It is a physiological adaptation of a person to the ETOH/Poly Sub that creates acute distress and intense cravings when the abuse stops.
    a. **Addictive**
    b. Progressive
    c. Problem Drinking
15. When an illness progresses in predicable stages and if not treated will result in irreversible dysfunction and eventually death. Increased dependence or loss of control can progress over a period of 5 to 15 years.
    a. Problem Drinking
    b. **Progressive**
    c. Chronic Alcoholism

16. Is an all-inclusive term which can include non- addictive ETOH behavior. An example would be driving an automotive while under the influence of ETOH. Or engaging in self destructive behavior (unprotected sexual behavior or altercations with strangers) while under the influence of ETOH.
    a. **Problem Drinking**:
    b. Chronic Alcoholism
    c. Steady Drinker with Binges
17. An advanced stage in the illness where severe medical or psychiatric complications occur.
    a. **Chronic Alcoholism**
    b. Steady Drinker with Binges
    c. Periodic Alcoholic
18. Is the degree of personal or social disintegration a person has to experience before they seek outside help for the addiction:
    a. Plateau Alcoholic
    b. **High or Low Bottom Alcoholics**
    c. Recreational Drunkenness
19. Usually includes psychological problems that are present prior to the person abusing and becoming dependent on ETOH. ETOH is often utilized for its psychological pain numbing effects.
    a. Low Bottom Alcoholic
    b. **Soil of Addiction**
    c. Pre-Alcoholics
20. Learned social and cultural behaviors may be a contributing factor. For example in Ireland and France there is a higher rate of ETOH abuse compared to other countries.
    a. **Sociocultural**
    b. Spiritual
    c. Both
    d. None of the above

21. Religious anxiety, fear of death, meaninglessness, unresolved guilt may contribute to ETOH abuse. Spiritual ETOH can falsely serve as a spiritual transcendences. ETOH addiction may serve as a form of idolatry.

    a. Sociocultural

    b. Spiritual

    c. Both

    d. None of the above

22. Sexual addiction is a serious problem in which one engages in persistent and escalating patterns of sexual behavior despite increasing negative consequences to one's self or others.

    a. True

    b. False

23. Approximately 300,000 children are at risk of being prostituted in the United States.

    a. True

    b. False

24. Up to 24 million people of all ages and genders suffer from an eating disorder (anorexia, bulimia and binge eating disorder) in the U.S.

    a. True

    b. False

25. Type 2 diabetes usually develops gradually over a number of years, beginning when muscle and other cells stop responding to insulin. This condition, known as insulin resistance, causes blood sugar and insulin levels to stay too low long after eating.

    a. True

    b. False

26. Diabetes remains the 7th leading cause of death in the United States in 2010, with 69,071 death certificates listing it as the underlying cause of death, and a total of 234,051 death certificates listing diabetes as an underlying or contributing cause of death.
    a. **True**
    b. False
27. 15.9% of this ethic group are diagnosed with diabetes
    a. Asian Americans
    b. Hispanics
    c. Non-Hispanic Black
    d. **American Indians/Alaskan Natives**
28. 13.2% of this ethic group are diagnosed with diabetes.
    a. Asian Americans
    b. Hispanics
    c. **Non-Hispanic Black**
    d. American Indians/Alaskan Natives
29. Annual Cost of Diabetes is:
    a. **$245 billion:**
    b. $176 billion
    c. $69 billion

30. In the brain, pleasure has a distinct signature: the release of the neurotransmitter _____ in the **nucleus accumbens**, a cluster of nerve cells lying underneath the cerebral cortex.
    a. Gluconate
    b. Norepinephrine
    c. **Dopamine**
    d. Serotonin

31. According to the current theory about addiction, **dopamine** interacts with another neurotransmitter _____ to take over the brain's system of reward-related learning.
    a. **Gluconate**
    b. Norepinephrine
    c. Dopamine
    d. Serotonin

32. Repeated exposure to an addictive substance or behavior causes nerve cells in the **nucleus accumbens** and the_____ (the area of the brain involved in planning and executing tasks) to communicate in a way that couples liking something with wanting it, in turn driving us to go after it.
    a. Brain Stem
    b. Prefrontal Cortex
    c. Hippocampus
    d. Cerebral Cortex
33. Addictive drugs, for example, can release _____the amount of **dopamine** that natural rewards do, and they do it more quickly and more reliably. In a person who becomes addicted, brain receptors become overwhelmed.
    a. 1 to 3 times
    b. 4 to 6 times
    c. 2 to 10 times
    d. 7 to 11 times.
34. The human brain utilizes glucose (fuel/energy) and water (oxygen) to function. Glucose comes from carbohydrate foods. Carbohydrates are made up of complex sugars (vegetables, grains, cereals) and simple sugars (fruits, juice, milk). A depletion or abuse in any of these resources will result in:
    k. Poor cognition
    l. Inattention
    m. Memory problems/loss
    n. Cell damage or cell death.
    o. All the Above
    p. None of the Above
35. Amino acids are the building block for many neurotransmitters.
    a. True
    b. False

36. Three amino acids that work with neurotransmitters are:
    a. Trypophan
    b. Taurine
    c. Tyrosine
    d. All the above
    e. None of the above

37. Neurotransmitters (help transport information through nerves) and proteins. They consist of:
    a. Dopamine, Serotonin,
    b. Norepinephrine, Epinephrine,
    c. Histamine. Dopamine
    d. All the above
    e. None of the above

38. _____gives the body a natural "high" when something good happens (sexual activity, exercise, achievements, etc). It is depleted by processed sugar, caffeine, alcohol, sleep deprivation, and some anti-depressants).
    a. Dopamine
    b. Serotonin
    c. Norepinephrine
    d. Epinephrine

39. _____ helps maintain mood levels, regulate the gastral intestinal track. It is depleted by alcohol, caffeine, nicotine, poor sunlight, exposure to heavy metals and pesticides. If elevated it can result in manic, psychotic behavior.
    a. Dopamine
    b. Serotonin
    c. Norepinephrine
    d. Epinephrine

40. _____it helps suppress neuro inflammation, regulated glucose release, and regulated the endocrine system. It is responsible for fight/flight response, attention response, decision making and goal directed behavior.
   a. Dopamine
   b. Serotonin
   c. Norepinephrine
   d. Epinephrine

41. _____its depletions can result in low blood pressure, excessive salt through kidneys, weight loss and chronic fatigue. What helps is sea salt and exercise.
   a. Dopamine
   b. Serotonin
   c. Norepinephrine
   d. Epinephrine

42. _____it maintains vigilance and alertness. Elevated levels found in people suffering from schizophrenia. It is naturally found in meats and hard cheeses.
   a. Serotonin
   b. Norepinephrine
   c. Epinephrine
   d. Histamine.

43. Refined Sugars reduce food nutrients and aggravates food intolerances.
   a. True
   b. False

44. Food Dyes contribute to AHDA behaviors and allergies in children.
   a. True
   b. False

45. The _____ and the _____ store information about environmental cues associated with the desired substance, so that it can be located again.
  a. **Hippocampus, Amygdala**
  b. Amygdala, Cerebral Cortex
  c. Prefrontal Lobe, Cerebral Cortex
  d. None of the Above
46. Whenever the person encounters_____. A person addicted to heroin may be in danger of relapse when he sees a hypodermic needle.
  a. Thoughts
  b. Feelings
  c. Environmental cues
  d. None of the above
47. Utilization of medical detoxification regime (in patient medical facility) that may be a few days until the patient is stabilized. Assign a psychiatrics or internal medicine physician to administer medication management with nursing care. Then given a social worker or case manager to plan after care treatment is called:
  a. Medical Intervention
  b. Psychological/ Behavioral Health Intervention
  c. Social workers and Case Managers
  d. Community of Faith
48. They are assigned a mental health counselor or psychologist for one on one treatment. Work on the behavioral and emotional factors that contribute to the compulsive addictive behavior. These sessions can be three to eight meetings. It also depends the philosophical orientation of the therapist. Some relationships may continue for a few years describes:
  a. Medical Intervention
  b. Psychological/ Behavioral Health Intervention
  c. Social workers and Case Managers
  d. Group Therapy

49. Due to the severity of the addictive process on their interpersonal relationships. They will need considerable assistance in basic living sustenance. May become indigent and homeless or have dependent children who need care and assistance. Many are unemployed, disabled or considered un employable due to criminal backgrounds. They are in need of considerable social assistance describes:
    a. Medical Intervention
    b. Psychological/ Behavioral Health Intervention
    c. Social workers and Case Managers
    d. Community of Faith
50. Support groups ran by professional clinicians with the same goals as individual counseling but with a greater focus on psychological educational materials are called:
    e. Medical Intervention
    f. Psychological/ Behavioral Health Intervention
    g. Social workers and Case Managers
    h. Group Therapy
51. A community organized around a common belief, creed, philosophical mindset or covenant. They provide counseling or pastoral care services to members of their particular community is called:
    e. Psychological/ Behavioral Health Intervention
    f. Community of Faith
    g. Group Therapy
    h. Self-Help Groups
52. These groups are directed by nonprofessionals and peers. Typically, the leaders are folks who have recovered or in the process of recovering from addictive disorders.
    a. Psychological/ Behavioral Health Intervention
    b. Community of Faith
    c. Group Therapy
    d. Self-Help Groups
53. Which definition is part of the Oxford Group's Five C's:
    a. Confidence
    b. Confession
    c. Conversion
    d. Continuance
    e. All the above

54. The Big Book of Alcoholics Anonymous in 1938 was founded by:
    a. Colonel Sanders
    b. Eleonore Roosevelt
    c. Bill Wilson
    d. W.C. Fields
55. The 12-Step Program itself is over_____ old,
    a. 20
    b. 50
    c. 70
    d. 100
56. We admit we are powerless over (addiction)—that our lives have become unmanageable is Step:
    a. 1
    b. 2
    c. 3
    d. 4
57. We make a decision to turn our will and our lives over to the care of God as we understand Him is Step:
    a. 1
    b. 2
    c. 3
    d. 4
58. We come to believe that a Power greater than ourselves can restore us to sanity is Step:
    a. 1
    b. 2
    c. 3
    d. 4
59. We admit to God, to ourselves, and to another human being the exact nature of our **wrongs is Step:**
    a. 5
    b. 6
    c. 7
    d. 8
60. We humbly ask Him to remove our shortcomings is Step:
    a. 5
    b. 6
    c. 7

d. 8

61. We make a searching and fearless moral inventory of ourselves is Step:
    a. 2
    b. 3
    c. 4
    d. 5

62. We make direct amends to such people wherever possible, except when to do so would injure them or others is Step:
    i. 9
    j. 10
    k. 11
    l. 12

63. We seek through prayer and <u>meditation</u> to improve our conscious contact with God as we understand Him, praying only for knowledge of His Will for us and the power to carry that out is Step:
    a. 9
    b. 10
    c. 11
    d. 12

64. We are entirely ready to have God remove all these defects of character is Step:
    a. 5
    b. 6
    c. 7
    d. 8

65. Having had a spiritual awakening as the result of these steps, we try to carry this message to alcoholics, and to practice these principles in all our affairs.
    a. 9
    b. 10
    c. 11
    d. 12

66. We continue to take personal inventory and when we are wrong promptly admitted it is step:
    m. 9
    n. 10
    o. 11

p. 12

67. We make a list of all persons we have harmed, and become willing to make amends to them all.
    a. 5
    b. 6
    c. 7
    d. 8

www.ingramcontent.com/pod-product-compliance
Lightning Source LLC
Chambersburg PA
CBHW060358190526
45169CB00002B/659